NEW DEVELOPMENTS IN MEDICAL RESEARCH

EVIDENCE-BASED MEDICINE AND PRACTICES

PRINCIPLES, IMPLEMENTATION AND EFFECTIVENESS

NEW DEVELOPMENTS IN MEDICAL RESEARCH

Additional books in this series can be found on Nova's website under the Series tab.

Additional e-books in this series can be found on Nova's website under the e-book tab.

NEW DEVELOPMENTS IN MEDICAL RESEARCH

EVIDENCE-BASED MEDICINE AND PRACTICES

PRINCIPLES, IMPLEMENTATION AND EFFECTIVENESS

ROSS T. BARNETT
EDITOR

NOVA BIOMEDICAL

New York

Library of Congress Cataloging-in-Publication Data

ISBN: 978-1-63482-362-3
Library of Congress Control Number: 2015937674

Published by Nova Science Publishers, Inc. † New York

Contents

Preface

In this book, an evidence-based approach to dietary and lifestyle medicine is taken. An approach known as "epidemiology-based health promotion," which compiles and presents available evidence that could help physicians, other healthcare professionals and members of the general public make wiser decision about healthcare, is also explored. Within this book, evidence-based practice (EBP) literature is reviewed, including literature on leadership and ethics in the field of internal medicine (compared to surgery) and how they affect the adoption of evidence-based medicine (EBM). A four-stage iterative model to identify procedures for implementing evidence based practices into applied settings is reviewed. The authors of the final chapter compare the cost-benefit and cost-effectiveness of all types of evidence-based medicine, both pharmaceuticals and non-drug complementary and alternative medicine (CAM) for all clinical conditions.

Chapter I – The current approach to evidence-based medicine was developed for the purpose of helping physicians make use of the vast amount of research that had started to come from the pharmaceutical industry, as a result of stricter regulation. Thus, it focuses almost exclusively on clinical trials, especially those with randomization, placebo controls, and blinding. However, this kind of focus is impractical for evaluating nutrition and lifestyle interventions, which seldom lend themselves to randomization or blinding and often take many years to show the intended effect. For that reason, an evidence-based approach to dietary and lifestyle medicine must take a broader view of the available evidence, including epidemiologic evidence. One promising approach would be to organize the available evidence according to the considerations suggested in 1965 by Sir Austin Bradford Hill for evaluating whether cigarette smoking causes lung cancer. By compiling and presenting the available evidence, epidemiologists could help physicians, other healthcare professionals, and members of the general public make wise decisions about healthcare and health promotion. This approach could be called epidemiology-based health promotion.

Chapter II – The authors review the evidence-based practice (EBP) literature to describe a universal design model that guides evidence based practice through an iterative process by providing standards and quality criteria for each of four different stages. They briefly review the history of EBP across different disciplines and discuss the consistency across these disciplines with respect to the guidelines, standards, and quality criteria used to determine the best practices based on evidence. The authors propose a four-stage iterative model, which consists of generating data from individual studies, aggregating data across multiple studies, synthesizing the strengths and weaknesses of aggregated data into generalizable treatment plans, and identifying procedures for implementing evidence based practices into applied settings, and suggest that these stages are common to all models of EBP. They describe how the findings within each of these stages are supported by previous research and collectively improve the EBP process. The authors conclude by discussing five ways that their model supports best practices, advances new research, and improves theory in an iterative manner.

Chapter III – Background: Leadership, ethics and the adoption of evidence-based medicine (EBM) are interrelated components of modern medical care. In today's medical world, cost-effectiveness, patient safety and outcomes are paramount. EBM is at the forefront while engrained medical traditions are scrutinized at an increasing rate. This shift in paradigm requires strong leadership. With this complicated arrangement, exploration and comparison of the concepts of leadership, ethics, and EBM in two prominent areas of healthcare, general internal medicine and surgery, is a valuable exercise. Objective: The primary objective of this work is to review the literature on leadership and ethics in the field of internal medicine compared to surgery and examine how they affect the adoption of EBM. The secondary objective is to identify aspects of leadership, ethics, and the implementation of EBM within internal medicine and surgery that may serve to improve the other discipline. Design: A review of the literature using Pubmed and Embase was performed. Keywords included leadership in internal medicine, leadership in surgery, ethics in internal medicine, ethics in surgery, evidence-based medicine in internal medicine, and evidence-based medicine in surgery. Setting: The Commonwealth Medical College, Scranton, PA. Results/Conclusion: The study identifies multiple similar qualities of leadership in internal medicine and surgery, especially the broad use of transformational leadership. While the less tangible qualities of charisma and personality are recognized, leaders who are willing to educate colleagues and work to solve problems with the healthcare system are required to generate acceptance of EBM by a healthcare team. Differences in leadership style that might affect the adoption of EBM exist between internal medicine and surgery. Internal medicine depends more on the culture of the team, while surgery depends more on the influence of powerful individual leaders. Other differences included internal medicine's greater appreciation for patient participation in care while surgical leaders are acknowledged most for technical skill and the ability to teach. Notably, both internal medicine and surgery ethical leaders refrain from conflicts of interest, especially regarding the increasing financial responsibilities, in order to maintain personal morals and the trust and respect of their healthcare teams. Ethical leaders in internal medicine place the patient's autonomy above the decisions of the medical team. Ethical leaders in surgery make appropriate decisions regarding heroic and end-of-life care. There are inherent differences between internal medicine and surgery that challenge the cross-over of leadership qualities from one discipline to the other. However, the differences in leadership style that do exist provide potential areas of improvement for each.

Chapter IV – *Aim*: To compare cost-benefit and cost-effectiveness of all types of evidences-based medicine, both pharmaceuticals and non-drug CAM for all clinical conditions. *Method*: Calculating therapeutic value ($TV=NNH_{total}/NNT$) and cost per cured patient (year 1-50) for 10 different types of evidence-based medicine. Cost is presented as EURO per cured patient, EURO per QALY, EURO per HALY, and number of harmed and killed patients per cured patient. The cost of one year of treatment was set to 2,000€, and the difference between healthy and sick to 20% (quality of life, self-rated health). *Results*: The authors found the most effective CAM-types (mind-body medicine, holistic medicine, shamanism) to be 100 times as cost-effective and 10.000 times less harmful compared to pharmaceuticals. The 50 years estimated cost for one patient cured was for: drugs 1,000,000€; physical therapy 100,000€; psychotherapy 100,000€; mind-body medicine 50,000€; holistic mind-body medicine 20,000€; one-session shamanistic healing with hallucinogenic drugs 2,000€. CAM is more efficient than drugs and has no side effects and adverse events, whereas treatment with drugs always has adverse effects and events. Only chemical medicine has mortality as adverse effect. *Interpretation*: To be useful medicine must have significant Therapeutic value (good ratio of benefits to harm: $TV \geq 1$) and documented long term effect and safety. The shift from drugs to CAM would improve health and quality of life radically in society and reduce harm to patients and the cost of healthcare to a small fraction. Strict laws should be introduced immediately in all countries to stop the pharmaceutical industry from promoting drugs without Therapeutic value, and from repressing CAM.

In: Evidence-Based Medicine and Practices
Editor: Ross T. Barnett
ISBN: 978-1-63482-362-3

Chapter I

An Evidence-Based Approach to Dietary and Lifestyle Medicine

Laurie Endicott Thomas*[*], *MA, ELS
Madison, NJ, US

Abstract

The current approach to evidence-based medicine was developed for the purpose of helping physicians make use of the vast amount of research that had started to come from the pharmaceutical industry, as a result of stricter regulation. Thus, it focuses almost exclusively on clinical trials, especially those with randomization, placebo controls, and blinding. However, this kind of focus is impractical for evaluating nutrition and lifestyle interventions, which seldom lend themselves to randomization or blinding and often take many years to show the intended effect. For that reason, an evidence-based approach to dietary and lifestyle medicine must take a broader view of the available evidence, including epidemiologic evidence. One promising approach would be to organize the available evidence according to the considerations suggested in 1965 by Sir Austin Bradford Hill for evaluating whether cigarette smoking causes lung cancer. By compiling and presenting the available evidence, epidemiologists could help physicians, other healthcare professionals, and members of the general public make wise decisions

[*] E-mail: laurie@gorillaprotein.com.

about healthcare and health promotion. This approach could be called epidemiology-based health promotion.

Evidence-Based Medicine and Pharmaceuticals

The main purpose of medical research is to guide medical decision-making. In 1972, a Scottish physician named Archibald Leman Cochrane pointed out that physicians were basing many treatment decisions on tradition or supposition because many widely accepted medical treatments had never been evaluated in randomized, controlled trials. [1] Cochrane made those observations at a time when the US Food and Drug Administration was starting to demand well-designed and well-run randomized, controlled clinical trials of efficacy and safety before it approved a new drug. [2] Regulatory agencies in other countries also established similar requirements. Because of these requirements, pharmaceutical companies conducted many high-quality studies of their new drug products. As a result, an enormous number of high-quality randomized controlled trials of pharmaceutical products were conducted, and many of these studies were published.

To help physicians make use of this growing body of evidence, much of it valuable, the Cochrane Collaboration was founded in 1993. [3] Participants in this nonprofit, international, nongovernmental organization conduct systematic reviews of the available research. Individual studies are rated according to the quality of their methodology. Well-designed double-blind, randomized controlled trials are given the highest rating. Yet even these "gold standard" studies have important scientific limitations [4]:

- They are generally too small to reveal some rare but potentially serious side effects.
- They do not last long enough to provide evidence of long-term efficacy and safety.
- They do not necessarily compare the treatment of interest to the best currently known approach, such as appropriate dietary management, for managing the problem being studied.

Often, a "gold standard" study cannot be done, for practical reasons, or should not be done, for ethical reasons. [4] For example, subjects cannot be blinded to their diet, and it would be unethical to assign subjects to an intervention or to a placebo treatment that is expected to result in serious harm without hope of benefit. In those situations, physicians and the general public must rely on other kinds of evidence.

By focusing only on randomized controlled trials, the conventional approach to evidence-based medicine could inadvertently bias physicians in favor of drug treatments and against dietary interventions, even for diseases that are known to be dietary in origin. [4] This problem is particularly serious given the general neglect of nutrition and dietetics in medical training [5-9].

Influence of the Tobacco Industry

Evidence-based medicine, as it is currently envisaged, could be reinforcing a form of bias that was promulgated by the tobacco industry in the mid 20th century. In 1957, the British Medical Research Council published a report that concluded that cigarette smoking is an important cause of lung cancer. [10] In response, the tobacco industry hired the brilliant statistician and geneticist Sir Ronald Aylmer Fisher to debunk the underlying studies. Fisher's arguments boiled down to the complaint that the epidemiologic studies merely established correlation, and that correlation does not prove causality. [11] Thus, Fisher cast unreasonable doubt on the conclusion that men and women could dramatically reduce their risk of getting lung cancer if they abstained from smoking cigarettes.

Fisher was one of the founders of the field of population genetics, and his work as a statistician laid the groundwork for the use of statistics in modern biology and medicine. Not only did he invent many important statistical methods, such as analysis of variance, but he wrote a practical handbook for researchers on how to design their studies and apply statistical analysis to the results. [12] Yet his efforts as a propagandist for the tobacco industry have cast a long shadow. His pro-tobacco rhetoric encouraged physicians to turn a blind eye to any study that does not follow the same methodology as a pivotal clinical trial for a drug product. His influence encouraged physicians to wait for a single, definitive study rather than taking a broad view of a body of evidence, in which the strengths of some studies compensate for the weaknesses of others.

Since then, other industry spokesmen and –women have used similar rhetorical tactics to sow similar confusion about such issues as the health effects of second-hand tobacco smoke, the environmental effects of acid rain, the effect of halocarbons on the ozone layer, and the role of the use of fossil fuels in promoting global warming. [13] The intent of these tactics was to confuse the general public and policymakers, thus undermining support for policies to protect public health and the environment [13].

Establishing Causality in Epidemiology

In response to Fisher's work for the tobacco lobby, Sir Austin Bradford Hill proposed an approach for using epidemiologic studies for establishing causality. [14] Although Hill was also a major proponent of randomization for assigning treatments in clinical trials, he recognized that physicians often must make decisions when no randomized clinical trial can or should be done. Hill listed some considerations—he did not consider them to be strict criteria—that can be applied in such situations (Table 1). [14] Hill did not advocate a formulaic approach. Instead, he wanted to emphasize wise and rational consideration of all of the available evidence.

The FDA generally requires 2 adequately designed randomized, controlled studies before it approves a new medicinal product or a new indication for an existing product. However, it accepted a single study with historical controls for the approval of lepirudin, a blood thinner that was used to treat a rare and potentially catastrophic disorder called type 2 heparin-associated thrombocytopenia. A randomized, controlled trial would have been unethical because there was no viable alternative treatment to use as a comparator. [15] All of the subjects in the trial were treated with lepirudin, and the results were compared with the data from earlier cases of type 2 heparin-associated thrombocytopenia.

Hill recognized that physicians did not need to wait for randomized controlled studies of cigarette smoking to establish whether cigarette smoking causes lung cancer. Such studies would, in fact, never be done because they would be not only impractical but unethical. Fortunately, by the late 1950s, there was already enough evidence for a reasonable person to accept the conclusion that the statistical relationship between cigarette smoking and lung cancer represented a causal relationship [10].

Table 1. Hill's Considerations for Evaluating Causality in Epidemiology [14]

Consideration	Explanation
Strength	Although correlation does not prove causality, the lack of correlation helps to rule out causality. A causal relationship is particularly likely when the statistical relationship between 2 variables is strong.
Consistency	If a causal relationship exists, then evidence of the statistical relationship should appear in studies conducted in different settings and with different methods.
Specificity	Is the environmental factor correlated with all-cause mortality or specifically with mortality from a particular cause? "If specificity exists we may be able to draw conclusions without hesitation; if it is not apparent, we are not thereby necessarily left sitting irresolutely on the fence." [14]
Temporality	A cause must always precede its effects.
Biological gradient	If a causal relationship exists, then individuals who have had more exposure to the cause generally have a higher incidence of the effect. Similarly, the incidence of a condition should decrease when its cause is reduced or eliminated.
Plausibility	The presumed causal relationship should be consistent with the currently accepted understanding of pathological processes. (Of course, research findings that conflict with established theory could lead to revision of the theory.)
Coherence	The underlying theory should be consistent with existing theory or knowledge. What other theories would have to be discarded in order for the causal relationship to be accepted?
Experiments	If some preventive action is taken because of an observed statistical association, does it in fact prevent the problem? Hill noted that experimental or even "semi-experimental" evidence in this context can be compelling. [14]
Analogy	Do other, similar things have similar effects? Hill noted, "With the effects of thalidomide and rubella before us we would surely be ready to accept slighter but similar evidence with another drug or another viral disease in pregnancy." [14]

When randomized, controlled trials cannot or should not be done, physicians should make wise use of the evidence that does exist. In Hill's schema, experimental evidence can be useful but is not always essential. As Hill explained, "Occasionally it is possible to appeal to experimental, or semi-experimental, evidence. For example, because of an observed association some preventive action is taken. Does it in fact prevent? The dust in the workshop is reduced, lubricating oils are changed, persons stop smoking cigarettes. Is the frequency of the associated events affected? Here the strongest support for the causation hypothesis may be revealed." [14] Unfortunately, many physicians are inclined to dismiss such compelling semi-experimental evidence out of hand if it comes from a study that does not meet the same strict requirements (e.g., randomization, controls, or blinding) that drug studies generally must meet.

Toward Epidemiology-Based Health Promotion

Evidence-based medicine was developed to help physicians decide whether giving a patient a particular medicine is better than doing nothing at all, and occasionally to decide whether one medicinal product is better than another for a given indication. Yet evidence-based medicine, as it is currently structured, provides only limited guidance for helping physicians decide what kind of care would be best for a particular patient at a particular point in time. To remedy this problem, epidemiologists must find ways to help physicians and laymen make use of epidemiologic evidence, as well as experimental evidence. One possible approach could involve the compilation of a wiki (modeled on Wikipedia) with a page devoted to each particular question, such as the role of diet in causing multiple sclerosis. The wiki should provide citations and preferably links to the source material. Hill's considerations for establishing causality in epidemiology can be used as a starting point for organizing the presentation.

It takes a much more extensive research effort to establish the value of lifestyle interventions (e.g., a low-fat, plant-based diet for preventing and managing multiple sclerosis) than it takes to establish the value of a drug treatment. Yet this evidence can be compiled and reviewed in a way that will allow nonspecialists and even laymen to make sense of the existing evidence. Table 2 provides an overview of the kinds of studies, and how they relate to Hill's considerations.

The first section of an epidemiology-based health promotion report should allow space for published guidelines or other position papers issued by various experts or expert panels. Although these summaries are generally the last part of the presentation to be written, they can be provided at the beginning of the presentation, for convenience. The wiki format will allow editors to comment on the standing of those guidelines in the light of emerging evidence.

Table 2. Evidence to Support Decision-Making in Dietary and Lifestyle Medicine

Section	Content
Overviews	Reviews and consensus documents.
Published guidelines	Guidelines published by expert panels.
Review articles	Concise reviews of all aspects of diagnosis and management. This section should include articles that compile and analyze the existing epidemiologic, laboratory, and clinical studies and for assessing the coherence of the evidence, its biological plausibility, and the viability of alternative explanations.
General background	Articles that provide general knowledge of the disease state and the methods used to study it.
Background	Descriptions of the scope and history of the problem.
Definitions	Discussions and validations of case definitions.
Methodology	Explanations and validation of methods for measuring the variables under consideration.
Epidemiologic studies	Studies that help to establish temporality, strength, dose effect, consistency, and specificity of the relationship between a possible causative factor and its purported effect.
Interregional comparisons	Comparisons of populations between geographic regions (e.g., the Seven Countries Study and the China-Cornell-Oxford Project.
Intraregional comparisons	Comparisons between subgroups within a population, such as a comparison of the rate of heart disease among Seventh Day Adventists, as compared with the general population.
Migration studies	Migration studies are useful for evaluating the role of environment and diet, as opposed to genes, in causing a disease.
Cross-sectional studies	Studies in which exposure and disease status are measured for individuals within a given population at a given point in time.
Longitudinal studies	Studies in which researchers detect changes over time in the characteristics of a target population at both the group and individual level,
Case-control studies	Studies in which individuals with a condition are compared with matched subjects who do not have that condition.
Cohort study	Prospective or retrospective observational studies of a defined group of individuals.
Occupational studies	Studies that compare people with a particular occupation to the general public.
Laboratory studies	Nonclinical studies that help to establish the biological plausibility of a causal relationship.
In vitro studies	Studies of human or nonhuman cells involved in a disease process.
Animal models	Studies of the pathophysiology or treatment of a condition in animals that resembles the human disease. The value of the model depends on the degree of similarity to the human disease.
Clinical studies	Studies involving human subjects.
Interventional studies	Studies in which human subjects receive some sort of intervention. Such studies are useful for ruling out confounding variables and establishing the direction of causality, as well as for documenting the magnitude and speed of response to intervention.

The second section should provide space for general review articles: articles that provide a concise overview of many aspects of the pathophysiology and treatment of the condition. The wiki format would allow editors to comment on the quality of the reviews.

The epidemiology-based health promotion report should also devote a section to general background. This section should include links to the basic literature documenting the history and scope of the problem. For example, it should include literature explaining how multiple sclerosis was discovered and how it came to be recognized as an entity that is separate from other neurologic diseases and especially other demyelinating diseases.

The Definitions section should include literature on the case definitions that have been used in clinical research. The goal should be to help practicing physicians as well as patients and their families understand how the diagnosis of multiple sclerosis is made, and how cases are classified (e.g., as relapsing-remitting or primary-progressive). There should also be some discussion of how these diagnostic criteria relate to the inclusion criteria of clinical studies. Such discussions will enable the physician and patient to see what the results of the clinical trials imply for that patient.

The Methodology section should include links to publications describing the materials and methods used in studies of the disease in question. For example, this section should include articles on the validation of the imaging methods that are used for diagnosing MS and for evaluating the outcome of treatment in clinical trials. This section should also include articles on the validation of various rating instruments, such as the Extended Disability Status Scale (EDSS) and the Scripps Neurologic Rating Scale (SNRS), that have been used in studies of MS patients.

The Epidemiologic Studies section would include many different kinds of studies, organized under various subheads. The goal of the Epidemiologic Studies section is to establish the statistical relationship between some environmental or dietary factor and the incidence or prevalence of a disease. It would include studies that establish the existence and temporality of a relationship between a possible cause and its purported effect. It would address questions such as the dose effect and the consistency and specificity of the relationships.

When one is evaluating the epidemiologic studies, it is important to consider how the strengths of one study can compensate for the weakness of another study. For example, a disease that is found to have a limited geographic distribution could result from some environmental factor that is present at some locales but not in others. The classic example is malaria, whose geographical distribution is limited by the geographic range of its insect vector. However, dietary habits also tend to be linked to geography, and the populations in different locales can differ genetically.

Geographic studies established that the prevalence of MS is strongly connected with latitude, with Scandinavia having the highest prevalence. Yet even within Scandinavia, the incidence of new cases of MS and progression of existing cases has varied substantially with respect to geography and with respect to time. In Norway, MS was found to be far more prevalent in dairying villages in the interior than in coastal fishing villages. [16] The incidence of new cases dropped dramatically during World War II, when fats and animal protein were in short supply, only to rise again after the war. [17] These findings strongly suggest that diet plays a strong role in the etiology of MS. Note that studies of this kind are likely to reveal information that would not be obtained from doing a case-control study of individuals who are all eating a similar diet.

Laboratory studies include in vitro studies and animal models. For MS, laboratory studies suggested a possible mechanism by which a fatty meal could cause increases in blood viscosity that led to the development of the perivascular lesions that are important in the pathophysiology of MS [18].

The epidemiologic studies provided compelling evidence for the role of diet in promoting the development and progression of MS. In light of that evidence, Roy Swank began advising his patients to make sharp restrictions in their intake of dietary fats, especially saturated fats. He then compared the disease progression in the patients who followed his dietary advice with that in patients who did not. "Good dieters" had far lower all-cause mortality and MS-related mortality than did the patients who continued to eat a fatty diet [19-23].

Regrettably, the value of Swank's simple and inexpensive yet powerful approach to managing a catastrophic disease has not been embraced by the medical profession, presumably because Swank's dietary study was neither randomized nor blinded. Yet it would have been impossible to blind patients to their diet, and it would have been unethical to randomly assign some patients to continue to eat the diet that was likely to be responsible for causing irreparable damage to their nervous system. Studies of similar dietary interventions for reversing heart disease, [24, 25] managing type 2 diabetes, [26] and slowing the progression of prostate cancer [27] have similarly been largely overlooked, for the same reason. Yet if physicians had taken Hill's criteria to heart, they would have understood that even "semi-experimental" evidence should have been sufficient in that context. The epidemiologic studies had already provided persuasive evidence of the role of diet in promoting MS. Evidence that a dietary change altered the course of the disease should have been compelling.

The Need for Epidemiology-Based Healthcare

Evidence-based medicine has been a way to help physicians make use of the scientific research that has been produced by the pharmaceutical industry, particularly in regard to their new, branded drugs that still have a long patent life. Consequently, evidence-based medicine, as it is currently structured, provides results that are often well-aligned with the marketing messages of major pharmaceutical companies. Thus, the conclusions of evidence-based medicine reports have been used to promote the sales of some presumably beneficial, and highly profitable, products. In contrast, epidemiologic studies have often yielded results that pose a threat to major industries.

Epidemiologic studies often yield evidence suggesting that consumers should stop consuming some hazardous product or that manufacturers should abandon or alter some hazardous industrial practice. From industry's perspective, the fallout from these studies can be serious: decreased revenues, increased costs, and even legal liability. The fallout might not be limited to a particular company or industry. For example, the news that cigarette smoking was a major cause of lung cancer posed a threat not just to the tobacco companies but to the advertising industry and the commercial media, both of which derived substantial revenues from cigarette advertising. Epidemiologic data on the health risks of various foods and beverages pose a similar threat to those same interests today. Epidemiologic data on the health risks of environmental toxins pose a threat to other industries. Thus, it is hardly surprising that epidemiology-based health promotion has not been embraced by industry. Any organization that intends to host an epidemiology-based health promotion wiki must establish safeguards to ensure that the wiki does not become corrupted by industry.

To appreciate the need for epidemiology-based health promotion, in addition to the existing approach to evidence-based medicine, ask yourself a simple question. At what point should physicians have started urging their patients to stop smoking? Should they have started in the 1930s, when there was a sudden outbreak of lung cancer, almost exclusively in men who had been heavy cigarette smokers for at least 15 years? [28] Or should they have held off until 1957, when the British Medical Research Council made its report implicating cigarette smoking as a cause of lung cancer? [10] Or should they have waited until 1964, when the US Surgeon General published a landmark report on smoking and health? [29] Or should they be waiting still, because there is still no randomized controlled study of the kind that Fisher claimed was needed? With that in mind, ask yourself how long physicians should wait before telling their MS patients that their fatty diet is probably the trigger for their illness and that they would probably benefit if they stopped pulling that trigger?

Epidemiology-based health promotion could provide an evidentiary basis for many of the kinds of decisions about self-care that can provide dramatic decreases in the incidence and prevalence of the diseases that represent the major causes of death and disability in the United States. [30] In particular, it would help physicians and laymen come to the realization that the same dietary recommendations that help to prevent and arrest multiple sclerosis also help to arrest and reverse coronary artery disease [25] and slow the progression of various cancers [27].

Physicians may feel that it is easy to prescribe a medication but hard to persuade patients to make significant changes in their diet and lifestyle. However, many patients do take their physicians' advice about diet and lifestyle. [31] Physicians may feel that they do not have the time to devote to dietary counseling or to giving advice about smoking cessation. Of course, physicians can easily refer their patients to other healthcare providers, such as registered dietitians or to a smoking cessation program, for such counseling.

Physicians have an ethical obligation to tell their patients about how diet and lifestyle affect health. Starting at least in the 1930s, consumers had a right to know that cigarette smoking was implicated as a cause of lung cancer. Similarly, people today have a right to know how their dietary choices affect their health. As Ancel Keys put it, "People should know the facts. Then if they want to eat themselves to death, let them." [32].

References

[1] Cochrane AL. *Effectiveness and Efficiency: Random Reflections on Health Services.* London, UK: Nuffield Provincial Hospitals Trust; 1972.

[2] Junod SW. FDA and clinical drug trials. 2014; Food and Drug Administration Web site. Silver Spring, MD: US Food and Drug Administration. Available at: http://www.fda.gov/AboutFDA/WhatWeDo/History/Overviews/ucm304485.htm. Updated: July 7, 2014. Accessed January 10, 2014.
[3] History. 2013; Cochrane Collaboration Web site. London: UK. Available at: http://www.cochrane.org/about-us/history. Updated: January 12, 2013.
[4] Thomas LE. How evidence-based medicine biases physicians against nutrition. *Med. Hypotheses.* 2013;81(6):1116-1119.
[5] Lloyd JK. Nutrition and the training of doctors. *Proc. Nutr. Soc.* 1984;43(2):219-221.
[6] Council of Food and Nutrition. Nutrition teaching in medical schools. *JAMA.* 1963;183:955-957.
[7] Nelson ES. Nutrition instruction in Medical Schools—1976. *JAMA.* 1976;236(22):2534.
[8] Committee on Nutrition in Medical Education. *Nutrition Education in U.S. Medical Schools.* Washington, DC: National Academy Press; 1985.
[9] Adams KM, Lindell KC, Kohlmeier M, Zeisel SH. Status of nutrition education in medical schools. *Am. J. Clin. Nutr.* 2006;83(4):941S-944S.
[10] Medical Research Council's statement on tobacco smoking and cancer of the lung. *Lancet.* 1957;272(6983):1345-1347.
[11] Gundle KR, Dingel MJ, Koenig BA. 'To prove this is the industry's best hope': big tobacco's support of research on the genetics of nicotine addiction. *Addiction.* 2010;105(6):974-983.
[12] Fisher RA. *Statistical Methods for Research Workers.* Edinburgh, UK: Oliver & Boyd; 1925.
[13] Oreskes N, Conway EM. *Merchants of Doubt: How a Handful of Scientists Obscured the Truth on Issues from Tobacco Smoke to Global Warming.* New York, NY: Bloomsbury Press; 2010.
[14] Hill AB. The environment and disease: association or causation? *Proc. R. Soc Med.* 1965;58:295-300.
[15] Refludan [Lepirudin (rDNA)] Injection [drug approval package]. Food and Drug Administration Web site. 1998. Available at: http://www.accessdata.fda.gov/drugsatfda_docs/nda/98/20807_Refludan.cfm.
[16] Swank RL, Backer J. The geographic incidence of multiple sclerosis in Norway. *Trans Am. Neurol. Assoc.* 1950;51:274-275.

[17] Swank RL. Multiple sclerosis; a correlation of its incidence with dietary fat. *Am. J. Med. Sci.* 1950;220(4):421-430.

[18] Swank RL. Subcutaneous hemorrhages in multiple sclerosis. *Neurology.* 1958;8(6):497-498.

[19] Swank RL. Treatment of multiple sclerosis with low-fat diet. *AMA Arch. Neurol. Psychiatry.* 1953;69(1):91-103.

[20] Swank RL. Treatment of multiple sclerosis with low-fat diet; results of five and one-half years' experience. *AMA Arch. Neurol. Psychiatry.* 1955;73(6):631-644.

[21] Swank RL. Treatment of multiple sclerosis with low-fat diet: result of seven years' experience. *Ann. Intern. Med.* 1956;45(5):812-824.

[22] Swank RL. Treatment of multiple sclerosis with a low-fat diet. *J. Am. Diet Assoc.* 1960;36:322-325.

[23] Swank RL. Multiple sclerosis: twenty years on low fat diet. *Arch. Neurol.* 1970;23(5):460-474.

[24] Esselstyn CB, Jr. Updating a 12-year experience with arrest and reversal therapy for coronary heart disease (an overdue requiem for palliative cardiology). *Am. J. Cardiol.* 1999;84(3):339-341, A338.

[25] Ornish D, Scherwitz LW, Billings JH, et al. Intensive lifestyle changes for reversal of coronary heart disease. *JAMA.* 1998;280(23):2001-2007.

[26] Barnard ND, Cohen J, Jenkins DJ, et al. A low-fat vegan diet improves glycemic control and cardiovascular risk factors in a randomized clinical trial in individuals with type 2 diabetes. *Diabetes Care.* 2006;29(8):1777-1783.

[27] Ornish D, Weidner G, Fair WR, et al. Intensive lifestyle changes may affect the progression of prostate cancer. *J. Urol.* 2005;174(3):1065-1069.

[28] Witschi H. A short history of lung cancer. *Toxicol. Sci.* 2001;64(1):4-6.

[29] *Smoking and Health: Report of the Advisory Committee to the Surgeon General of the Public Health Service.* Washington, DC: Public Health Service.

[30] Xu J, Kochanek KD, Murphy SL, Tejada-Vera B. Deaths: Final Data for 2007. *Natl Vital Stat Rep.* 2010;58(19).

[31] Greenlund KJ, Giles WH, Keenan NL, et al. Physician advice, patient actions, and health-related quality of life in secondary prevention of stroke through diet and exercise. *Stroke.* 2002;33(2):565-570.

[32] The fat of the land. *Time.* January 13, 1961. Available at: http://www.time.com/time/magazine/article/0,9171,828721-8,00.html.

In: Evidence-Based Medicine and Practices
Editor: Ross T. Barnett
ISBN: 978-1-63482-362-3

Chapter II

Toward A Universal Design Model of Evidence-Based Practice

Gregory Schraw [1] and Erika A. Patall [2]
[1]Educational Psychology and Higher Education,
University of Nevada, Las Vegas, NV, US
[2]Educational Psychology,
The University of Texas at Austin, Austin, TX, US

Abstract

We review the evidence-based practice (EBP) literature to describe a universal design model that guides evidence based practice through an iterative process by providing standards and quality criteria for each of four different stages. We briefly review the history of EBP across different disciplines and discuss the consistency across these disciplines with respect to the guidelines, standards, and quality criteria used to determine the best practices based on evidence. We propose a four-stage iterative model, which consists of generating data from individual studies, aggregating data across multiple studies, synthesizing the strengths and weaknesses of aggregated data into generalizable treatment plans, and identifying procedures for implementing evidence based practices into applied settings, and suggest that these stages are common to all models of EBP. We describe how the findings within each of these stages are supported by previous research and collectively improve the EBP process. We conclude by discussing five ways that our model supports best practices, advances new research, and improves theory in an iterative manner.

Toward a Universal Design Model of Evidence-Based Practice

High quality data based on sound empirical research enables a discipline to improve theory and practice in the most effective manor (Bellamy, Bledsoe & Traube, 2006; Wilczynski, 2012). In a previous article (Schraw & Patall, 2013) in a special issue of *Educational Psychology Review*, we voiced concerns with the practice of providing recommendations for educational policy based on single investigations reported in primary research journals. We argued that primary research journals are well suited to publishing individual intervention studies with the highest possible degree of internal validity, but they are less well suited for offering recommendations for practice due to limited data within the scope of a single study (or set of studies in a single investigation) and separation from practice and policy experts. We suggested the use of a universal design, cyclical model with four stages to achieve the highest level of empirical support for evidence-based practices. In this paper, we extend this argument by describing four stages based on generating a data base from individual studies, data aggregation using meta-analytic procedures, synthesis of aggregated findings into treatment interventions, and systematic implementation and assessment of best practices in applied settings. Our model (see Figure 1) draws on previous iterative, systems-based frameworks (Brug, van Dale, Lanting, Kremers, Veenhof, Leurs, van Yperen and Kok, 2010; Carey, Buchan & Sanson-Fischer, 2009; Odom, Brantlinger, Gersten, Horner, Thompson & Harris, 2005; Schalock, Vedugo & Gomez, 2011) and extends them by focusing on the four stages common to all of them. The intent of our model is to describe an iterative, universal design process that illustrates how quality data informs subsequent best-practice decisions, which in turn leads to additional research and the further development of theory.

We believe it is important to develop a universal model that offers sound guidelines to researchers and practitioners in a variety of clinical disciplines such as education, mental health, and medicine. Our main argument is that good practice does not always follow directly from good research, but is mediated by syntheses of findings and thoughtful implementation of documented practices based on well-controlled research that has been carefully evaluated by clinicians and practitioners to maximize its contextual utility (Carey et al., 2009). Like others, we believe that recommendations should be based on aggregated data within coherent programs of research that are most likely to approximate real-world settings using the *logic-of-generalization* guidelines proposed by Shadish (1995).

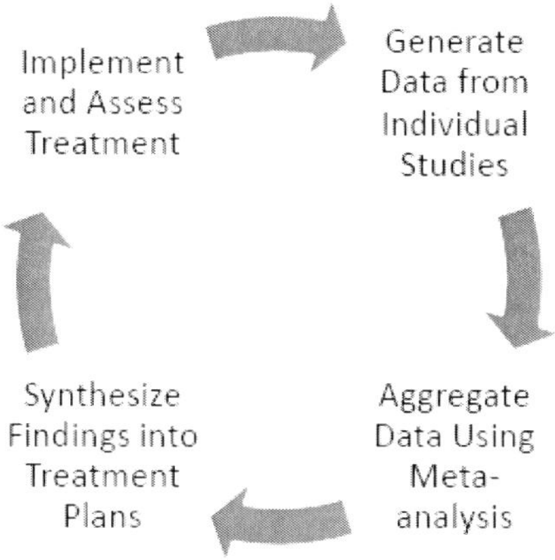

Figure 1. A Four-Stage Universal Design Model of Evidence-Based Practice.

This article is divided into three sections that describe the model in Figure 1. The first section provides a backdrop to EBP in which we briefly discuss the development of EBP and three key foundational assumptions. Section two summarizes components of the four-stage iterative model, including the evaluative criteria used for collecting, assessing, implementing and evaluating research findings and treatment interventions. We argue that each step in the sequence involves a different stakeholder group in which diverse views and values impact decision making. Section three considers five advantages of the model.

Overview of EBP Principles

Evidence based practice refers to a process in which a hierarchy of evidence based on the soundness of experimental methods is used by panels of experts to make the best possible clinical decisions (Chorpita, Bernstein & Daleiden, 2011; Dozois, 2013; Linkov, Welle, Loney, Tkachuk, Canis, Kim, & Bridges, 2011; Slavin, 2008). Central to this view, existing archival research have focused primarily on syntheses of individual studies into meta-analyses that provide the basis for EBP suggestions (Jenson, Clark, Kircher & Kristjansson, 2007). Although researchers agree that EBP is attainable, a number of recent reviews have identified a *research-to-practice gap* that sometimes impedes it (Dozois, 2013; Cook, Smith & Tankersley, 2012s). Namely, even after identifying best practice based on current research evidence, disparities between applied practice in clinical or educational settings and findings from research on field-based effectiveness often remain due to the reluctance of scholars and practitioners to base practices on research that is inconsistent or highly nuanced in its conclusions (Cook et al., 2012). Moreover, three procedural problems are endemic to this approach, including the assumption that the results of individual studies typically were replicable, that aggregated results provided the best overall EBP delivery strategy, and the under-utilization of task forces to contextualize general findings to accommodate real-world constraints (Bellamy et al., 2006; Chorpita et al., 2011; Drotar, 2010). Recent EBP initiatives have strived to close the gap between data-based recommendations and implementation of a treatment in classroom settings.

Cook et al. (2012, p. 498) considered three claims that provide the logical foundation for EBP. One is that scientific research is the most reliable method for determining effective instructional practices and programs. This is reflected in the movement in federally funded research programs, as well as increased methodological rigor as recommended by the What Works Clearinghouse (2008), that call for the use of controlled randomized studies. A second is that the most effective instructional practices and programs produce the highest student outcomes. This claim assumes that comparable high-quality studies may be analyzed collectively to identify the strongest effect sizes for a variety of clinical interventions, and that replicating the procedures used in these studies in applied settings will lead to significant improvement in the outcomes of target individuals in a majority of cases. A third is that practitioners can appropriately apply practices identified as effective by scientific research in local clinical and classroom settings. This claim assumes that treatment planning and implementation fidelity are high and perhaps guided by closely scripted intervention activities. Although not without important exceptions and limitations, these claims are largely regarded as valid by the scientific community. As such, it remains an important task for both the scientific and practitioner communities to have an effective process for identifying and applying EBPs.

Over the last decade, a number of advances have occurred in terms of identifying EBP models (Odom et al., 2005; Schalock et al., 2011), quality criteria for conducting and aggregating individual studies (Brug et al., 2010), guidelines for using aggregated data to develop treatment interventions, the development of treatment implementation rules, and guidelines for evaluating EBP that may lead to ongoing research studies and treatment planning (Carey et al. 2009; Jenson et al; 2007). We discuss each of these in greater detail below in the next section.

Overview of the Four-Stage Model

The model shown in Figure 1 includes four types of activities we refer to as generating data, aggregating data, synthesis of findings into systematic treatment intervention plans, and implementation of the treatment interventions with subsequent modifications if necessary. Table 1 summarizes core activities, primary research objectives, and use of quality criteria for assessing treatment effectiveness, key participants, and important challenges to the EBP process. A variety of guidelines have been proposed for planning a treatment intervention.

Table 1. Activities and Criteria within the Four-Stage Model of EBP

Stage	Core Activities	Purpose of Research	Quality Criteria	Key participants	Challenges
Stage 1: Generate data in laboratory and clinical settings.	Plan and execute theory-based studies that investigate the effectiveness of interventions.	Evaluate key theoretical premises and assumptions. Assess treatment effectiveness. Isolate cause (i.e., mechanism of change) of treatment effect.	Conduct theory-based intervention research. Maintain high methodological standards for treatment implementation and internal validity.	Researchers in a variety of laboratory and field settings examining a variety of plausible treatments.	Standardize the treatment. Conduct true experiments in authentic settings. Generalize from a single study.

Table 1. (Continued)

Stage	Core Activities	Purpose of Research	Quality Criteria	Key participants	Challenges
Stage 2: Aggregate data to evaluate intervention effects and moderating variables.	Conduct literature review; assess quality of each study; establish data base of effect sizes; conduct meta-analysis.	Estimate effect sizes of specific treatments. Disaggregate effect size as a function of moderating variables.	Technical merit of individual studies (internal validity); reliability of scores; statistical conclusion validity of meta-analysis.	Research synthesis teams.	Define target construct. Identify relevant studies. Categorize studies by treatment intervention and targeted population.
Stage 3: Synthesize findings to identify best practices within specific intervention contexts.	Experts assess the feasibility of interventions within different settings and articulate a theory of practice logic model.	Assess and compare the utility of treatments to the individual, the organization and to society.	Relevance of intervention. Optimize field-based utility (i.e., match intervention to situational constraints).	Researchers, policy experts, clinicians, and teachers	Establish clear criteria for EBP recommendations. Obtain agreement among diverse experts.
Stage 4: Implement and assess best practices in field settings.	Implement and assess interventions. Generate new research questions. Provide feedback.	Test a specific intervention. Collect formative and summative data. Provide feedback.	Standardizing treatments. Detailed implementation plan. Optimizing implementation fidelity. External validity.	Clinicians, teachers, evaluators.	Overcome potential barriers. Optimize treatment delivery and fidelity.

Stage 1: Generating Data

The main purpose of stage one activities is to generate data for individual studies using a common set of on discipline-wide criteria. To do so, researchers must plan and execute studies based on theory with a special emphasis on identifying a *mechanism of change* in the treatment intervention that improves target outcomes (Dozois, 2013). Brug et al. (2010, see Table 1) provided an extensive list of quality control criteria for planning individual studies to maximize the likelihood of treatment success and generalizability. Chief among these are specifying the theoretical framework that supports the study, identifying the short and long term goals of the intervention, implementing appropriate treatment timing given the goals of the intervention, ensuring a high-fidelity intervention, and outlining the expected costs of the intervention and its implementation. Jitendra, Burgess and Shigajria (2011) and Wilczynski (2012) also provide a review of similar quality criteria for planning treatments as well as assessing the methodological quality of individual studies. To meet the growing need to identify well-designed studies that produce trustworthy conclusions, many authors and governmental agencies also have proposed quality criteria guidelines for methodologically rigorous studies and created systems for evaluating the extent to which claims of an intervention's effectiveness are supported by rigorous research (e.g., What Works Clearinghouse, 2008; Blueprints for Violence Prevention, 2004; The National Registry of Evidence-Based Programs and Practices, 2007; Sherman & Gottfredson, 1997 [Maryland Scale]). These guidelines generally include situating research within a compelling theoretical framework (Carey et al., 2009; Chou, 2008a), sampling from both group and single subject research designs (Montague & Dietz, 2009, see Tables 1 and 2), design validity (Jitendra et al., 2011), the construct validity of research instruments and outcome variables (Cook et al., 2012), statistical reporting (Schalock et al., 2011), attrition (Chou, 2008a; Farmington, 2007),effect sizes and causal conclusions (Rubin & Parrish, 2007; Shadish, Cook & Campbell, 2002; Staines, 2008), and ease of implementation (Dozois, 2013).

Treatment fidelity is another important methodological constraint that has been considered in detail, especially with respect to treatment replication across participants and settings. Dozois (2013) recommended continuous assessment to measure outcomes on an ongoing basis in order to determine not only if a specific intervention is effective, but also it's changing trajectory over time. Three outcomes represent prototypical trajectories, including no change due to the treatment, a gradual linear change that is monotonic in nature, and a curvilinear change that may ebb and flow over the course of the intervention timeframe. Most authors suggest a multitrait/multimethod approach to accomplish these goals in which multiple outcome measures are administered at regular intervals over time to triangulate change due to treatment.

Treatment planning and delivery have been identified as important constraints on treatment effectiveness. Smith, Daunic and Taylor (2007) proposed a variety of recommendations both for treatment implementation and the assessment of treatment fidelity. Five strategies were used to document treatment fidelity, including selection of an appropriate theory, convening experts to plan the treatment (i.e., a treatment planning workgroup), training, treatment delivery schedules, and success of treatment enactment on the part of individuals trained to perform a skill or set of skills. Regarding the assessment component, Smith et al. (2007) outlined five common methods, including direct observation of each phase of treatment implementation, feedback from treatment providers and independent observers, self-monitoring and reporting from practitioners and participants during or after the intervention, review of permanent products, and treatment manualization, which specifies the level of skills participants are expected to master by the end of the intervention.

Perhaps no topic has been discussed more than the use of guidelines to evaluate the quality of evidence that is collected in individual studies. Krainovich-Miller, Haber and Jacobs (2009) described a seven-level rating system for the quality of evidence produced by different research designs ranging from randomized control designs based on aggregated effect sizes to personal opinions. A number of authors have proposed similar hierarchies, as has the What Works Clearhinghouse (2008), leading to strong agreement that randomized control studies (i.e., true experiments) exceed the quality of quasi-experiments and regression discontinuity designs (Imbens & Lemieux, 2008), which in turn exceed non-experimental (e.g., correlational and cohort studies), single subject designs, and qualitative studies. In response to the lack of quality criteria in empirical research (e.g., Jüni, Witshci, Bloch, & Egger, 1999; Valentine & Cooper, 2008), Valentine and Cooper (2008) designed a multilevel and hierarchical instrument based in the philosophical perspective of Donald Campbell (e.g., Shadish et al., 2002), the Study Design Implementation and Assessment Device (Study DIAD), that is designed to yield a profile of scores corresponding to the four classes of inferential validity (internal, external, measurement, and statistical) recognized throughout the social sciences (Shadish et al., 2002) to represent study quality.

Table 1 summarizes the main activities and challenges encountered in stage one. The goal of individual studies is to plan and execute theory-based studies that investigate the causal effects of the intervention. To do so, researchers must develop credible treatments within the broader context of a theoretical framework that describes potential causal mechanisms included in the treatment to improve important outcomes (Dozois, 2013) and to follow rigorous interpretative guidelines for making causal inferences (Shadish et al., 2002; Staines, 2008). There is widespread agreement that such studies should utilize randomized control trials whenever possible to isolate the effects of specific causes (Schneider, Carnoy, Kilpatrick, Schmidt & Shavelson, 2007). These studies tend to be undertaken by well-trained researchers in field settings. Some of the most significant challenges are to identify a theoretically justifiable treatment intervention, standardize the treatment protocol, conduct true experiments in authentic settings, and generalize findings from a single study.

Stage 2: Aggregating Data

Researchers agree that aggregated research findings based on an exhaustive sample of individual studies is superior with respect to estimating treatment-effects and replication probability. Indeed, Miller and Schwarz (2011) found that the replication probability of individual studies was so low, accurate estimates often are unattainable. Nevertheless, researchers likewise agree that aggregated data present inferential challenges due to differences in the research designs, participants, methods, data analysis, and treatment fidelity of constituent studies (Jenson et al., 2007), with some recent research revealing less than 50% of studies used in these analyses are of adequate methodological rigor (Rubin & Parrish, 2007). One special concern is the restricted nature of randomized trials that may limit findings due to the limited range and duration of interventions being tested (Westen & Bradley, 2005). However, some have argued that differences among individual studies, but especially methodological differences across studies, may be an asset, allowing the research synthesists to systematically explore heterogeneity in findings as a function of study differences through moderator analyses (Cooper, Hedges, & Valentine, 2009). Meta-analyses can reveal factors that may influence effects that have never been studied in a single study, but became apparent across studies. Second, meta-analyses in the social and medical sciences are often small, having relatively few studies meeting a priori inclusion criteria. This is especially true for those meta-analyses focused on research designs of most interest to EBPs, experimental and quasi-experimental research, because of the many challenges associated with conducting experimental research in applied settings. Half the meta-analyses in the Cochrane Library, for example, include 7 studies or fewer (Evangelou,

Ioannidis, & Patsopoulos, 2007) and a brief look at studies meeting standards for quality according to the What Works Clearinghouse (WWC) initiative of the Institute for Education Sciences (IES) at the U.S. Department of Education suggests that the extent of evidence includes less than 10 studies for most, if not all, education interventions. As a consequence, even detailed aggregated findings may not be methodologically adequate to warrant causal explanations of treatment effects (Fingeld-Connett, 2010; Schneider et al., 2007; Staines, 2008).

Other constraints in meta-analysis such as the researchers' theoretical backgrounds and study-selection/interpretation biases can be important contributors to the determination of intervention effectiveness as well (Schalock et al., 2011). For example, as Table 1 suggests, the validity of meta-analyses may be challenged to the extent that decisions about the relevance of studies to a topic may be influenced by factors such as the amount of information available about the study, researcher expertise, and criteria for research quality (see Valentine & Cooper, 2008). Nevertheless, even these concerns can be addressed by obtaining consensus on decisions across multiple judges, using an empirical a posteriori approach to assessing the impact of design and implementation variation (i.e., the impact of quality variation) on study results, specifying precise conceptual and operational definitions, and situating the problem to be addressed in the synthesis within a broader theoretical and practical context (see Cooper, 2010).

Chou (2008a, Tables 1-4) provided detailed criteria for evaluating the quality of aggregated data for use in EBP. These criteria focus on the advantages of systematic and quantitative data-based aggregation methods over narrative approaches to review (Chou's Table 1), criteria for evaluating syntheses (Table 2), criteria for assessing the quality of randomized trials (Table 3), and clinical guidelines for grading the quality of synthesized research evidence (Table 4). Collectively, the criteria summarized by Chou (2008a, b) and others (Cooper et al., 2011) provide a systematic process for gathering, aggregating, and interpreting a body of research in order to form (or intentionally not form) trustworthy recommendations for practice and policy.

Like quality criteria for generating data, there is cross-disciplinary agreement for evaluating the quality of research syntheses. Cooper (2007) specified 20 questions that could be asked concerning the validity of research synthesis conclusions. These include questions regarding the nature of the intervention, how the literature was searched and information was retrieved, the correspondence between methods and implementation of individual studies and the desired inferences in synthesis, the appropriateness and completeness of analysis methods, and whether sensitivity analyses were carried out. Regardless of the specific criteria used, the strength of aggregated data determines the extent to which intervention outcomes can be compared and prioritized for field-based trials. This claim is widely supported and illustrated by conceptual models in a number of recent discussions of EBP (Dozois, 2012, Krainovich-Miller et al., 2009; Schalock et al., 2011).

Stage 3: Synthesizing Findings from Aggregated Data into Systematic Treatment Plans

One of the most challenging endeavors in EBP is translating the results of meta-analyses into a strategic plan for implementing intervention-research findings into practice (Cook et al., 2012; Slavin, 2008). One reason is that treatment development requires a close collaboration between those who conduct and synthesize research, and those who use these results to improve treatment effectiveness in applied settings. Often these groups are not the same (Bellamy et al., 2006). One of the most effective ways to improve the treatment-development process is to utilize diverse panels with wide-ranging expertise in settings in which the treatment is implemented. Guidelines for how data might inform practices that incorporate the expertise of practitioners and policy-makers are summarized by Wecker (2013) to guide the research-to-practice sequence.

Chou (2008, b) likewise proposed three criteria to help clinicians select, implement, and assess the most effective interventions at their disposal:

1. Evaluate the applicability of aggregated results to clinical practice guidelines, including the closeness of the match to the sample, setting, and procedures of critical studies within the meta-analysis. Assess the extent to which all expert perspectives were represented
2. Identify criteria for both assessing the clinical effectiveness of interventions and considering the cost-benefit implications within specific clinical settings. Assure that guidelines remain current over time.
3. Specify the most likely clinical practice outcomes that the intervention program hopes to achieve. Ideally, these outcomes are expressed as specific objectives with respect to the kind or amount of outcome improvement.

It is important to note that these criteria are necessary but not sufficient. Carefully aggregated data presumably provides a reasonable account of treatment effectiveness for the interventions, samples, and settings captured in studies included in the synthesis, and often variation in treatment effectiveness. Nevertheless, insightful policy recommendations require more than researchers summarizing data in a reliable way and developing a plan for implementing and evaluating findings in practice.

One of the most important concepts discussed in the EBP literature is that of *relevance of evidence* to the treatment-development process. Schalock et al. (2011) proposed that both *evidence indicators* (e.g., physical, behavioral and psychological outcomes) and *evidence gathering strategies* (e.g., randomized trials, multiple baseline and single subject designs) must be relevant at the individual, organizational and societal levels. Data should be assessed at multiple points in time and compared using cross-sectional and longitudinal analyses. Schalock et al. (2011) also distinguished among three types of treatment effectiveness decisions that should be considered, including clinical decisions that affect individual clients, managerial decisions that affect the cost-benefit of interventions, and public policy decisions that affect the intervention's societal effectiveness. To assure relevance, two expertise-driven strategies have been proposed to select and implement EBPs when beliefs and values differ among researchers, policy makers and clinicians. Chorpita et al. (2011) developed a methodology referred to as *relevance mapping*, which allows individuals to make a structured comparison among multiple EBPs in order to select the most appropriate, utilitarian applied interventions. Linkov et al. (2011) described a similar procedure based on weight of evidence (WOE) risk assessment strategies in which stakeholders use multiple quantitative and qualitative lines of evidence in a collaborative manner to select candidate interventions. Both of these strategies help to make different stakeholder values and decision-making uncertainty more explicit, and therefore easier to address and resolve constructively (Dozois, 2012; Wilczynski, 2012). Nevertheless, as shown in Table 1, challenges exist with respect to establishing clear criteria for EBP recommendations and obtaining agreement among diverse experts.

Stage 4: Implementing and Assessing Treatment Plans

The real test of EBP research is to construct and implement treatments in the most rigorous manner possible. This may be difficult due to a number of *barriers* discussed in the literature, including lack of trust by teachers, resistance to school change, treatment diffusion in clinical settings, uncertainty as to whether treatments generalize to everyday settings, lack of treatment fit to individuals or setting, and insufficient resources that may undermine the effectiveness of the treatment intervention (Bellamy et al. 2006; Cook et al., 2012; Dozois, 2013).

Carey et al. (2008) developed a three-phase implementation process with 12 subcomponent steps. The three phases are: (1) identify best-practice guidelines; (2) develop an implementation plan; and (3) pilot test clinical strategies. The core activities across the three phases include identifying what the results of research studies suggest, identifying actionable field-based priorities, translating priorities into situationally specific action plans, engaging stakeholders in the utility of these plans, pilot testing, evaluating, and refining strategies. Because of the likely gap between researcher and stakeholder values, perhaps the most essential component is to assure practitioner "buy-in" through a careful justification of best practices (Schalock et al., 2011). This step is essential in educational practice because of a deep-seated value-gap between researchers, teachers, and the public (Hemsley-Brown & Sharp, 2003).

In addition, Chorpita et al. (2011) provided five general guidelines that are echoed throughout the EBP literature. One is to define the treatment carefully, including an explanation of its presumed causal effects, to help justify the use of a particular intervention over others. Second, construct a detailed treatment protocol that illustrates major events, timeframes and important measurable outcomes. Third, elicit administrative support for the project and meet with parents, teachers and other stakeholders to assuage distrust or lack of buy-in. Fourth, provide comprehensive training and consultation in advance of the intervention, clarifying important milestones and expected outcomes. Fifth, conduct formative and summative evaluations of the intervention and provide detailed feedback to all parties.

As shown in Table 1, stage four is likely to be more fraught with challenges than stages one through three, in part, due to the shift from conducting individual or aggregated studies to a working in a field setting where researchers are dependent upon clinical partners. One challenge is overcoming barriers. A second challenge is implementing the treatment with optimal fidelity. Research suggests the most effective strategy to reduce challenges is to follow the five guidelines described by Chorpita et al. (2011).

Five Advantages to Using an Iterative Multi-Stage Model

The goal of this chapter was to elaborate on a four-stage cyclical model of EBP. We believe there are five ways this model improves the research-to-practice endeavor. One is to identify four individual stages that are common to all types of EBP regardless of discipline. Table 1 refers to these as generating data, aggregating data, synthesizing findings and implementing and assessing treatments. Our review of the literature suggests that a variety of activities at each of these stages must occur to assure the best outcomes in applied settings. In addition, most disciplines have developed similar quality criteria to guide the evaluation of activities at each stage, but especially evaluating individual studies, the results of meta-analysis, and criteria for inferring causal effects between a treatment intervention and outcomes (Krainovich-Miller et al., 2009; Schneider et al., 2007; Shadish et al., 2002; Staines, 2008).

A second way our model improves EBP is by emphasizing the iterative nature of the research-to-practice cycle. Activities at each stage are important; however, these activities should provide both *forward* and *backward feedback* to researchers in terms of what kind of studies to conduct, how to select studies in order to aggregate findings, providing multiple perspectives on the importance of treatment interventions, and practical constraints that occur in field-based settings (Chou, 2008a, b). Realistically, best practices are most likely to occur after several rounds of data generation and field-testing of credible treatment interventions. Implicitly, the model in Figure 1 assumes that researchers are not engaged in a search for a single-best practice, but a process in which several possible treatments are potentially useful depending upon the specific constraints of the intervention context.

Third, the model likewise emphasizes the role of feedback in stage four for evaluating the effectiveness of treatments as well as generating new interventions. Each new study should advance practice and theory in some important way. We hope that a clear theory of action is generated in stage three that can be used to construct a logic model that justifies a particular intervention in stage four (Dozois, 2013). In turn, triangulated assessment data at stage four can be used to evaluate the treatment as well as the theory of action it is based on.

A fourth way the model advances research is to help researchers identify new types of data and strategies for weighting multiple sources of data that may be useful for evaluating an intervention (Linkov et al., 2011). A careful review of an intervention by the researchers may reveal types of data that were not collected that might be useful in future studies. Closely related is the idea that changes to the intervention itself in either the form of a new intervention or a hybrid adaption may improve its utility. We believe the transition from the implementation and assessment phase of one study to improved interventions, methods, or data collect in subsequent studies supports EBP to the extent it helps researchers better articulate a clear program of research based on a testable theory of action (Carey et al., 2009; Cook et al., 2012; Chou, 2008b; Dozois, 2013).

A fifth way the model promotes EBP is to build stronger relationships among researchers, policy experts, school administrators and teachers at stages three and four. Stages three and four explicitly call for interdisciplinary teams to design, implement and evaluate treatment interventions. These teams are especially well suited to assess the strengths and risks of intervention treatments (Wilczynski, 2012). All members of these interdisciplinary teams need to be involved in the selection and use of quality indicators to plan, implement and assess interventions. In addition, classroom teachers are perhaps best suited to judge the practical relevance of interventions and match the intervention to specific situational constraints (Chorpita et al., 2011; Cook et al., 2012; Jitendra et al., 2011).

Conclusion

Our discussion suggests that effective EBP is the end product of a multi-stage, iterative process that begins with valid and replicable empirical findings based on individual studies that are aggregated, evaluated by a multi-disciplinary team of experts, and parceled into tailored instructional guidelines (Krainovich-Miller et al., 2009). We believe it is naïve to assume that research findings from individual studies can be directly translated into generalizable practice because even if high-quality empirical results exist, the beliefs and methodological choices of experts during data-aggregation and codification stages may lead to differences of opinion regarding the educational value of various EBPs (Jenson et al., 2007). Moreover, the transition from implementation plans to stakeholder buy-in and field-based implementation likely represents the biggest fracture point within the four-stage sequence due to competing beliefs, worldviews about research and practice, and disparate values (Hemsley-Brown & Sharp, 2003). Notably, stage three of the model in

Figure 1 utilizes policy discussions and decisions based on inter-disciplinary teams of researchers, policy makers and practitioners (Carey et al., 2009; Chorpita et al., 2011; Chou, 2008, 2008b), while stage four specifies when and where different types of educational interventions are most effective in different situational contexts. We hope our model provides grist for more sophisticated models and that future studies evaluate the effectiveness of these models as planning and implementation tools.

References

Bellamy, J. L., Bledsoe, S. E., & Traube, D. E. (2006). The current state of evidence-based practice in social work: A review of the literature and qualitative analysis of expert interviews. *Journal of Evidence-Based Social Work, 3*, 23-48.

Blueprints for Violence Prevention. (2004). *Blueprints Model Programs Selection Criteria*. Retrieved August 17, 2014, from http://www.colorado.edu/cspv/blueprints/.

Brug, J., van Dale, D., Lanting, L., Kremers, S., Veenhof, C., Leurs, M., van Yperen, T., & Kok, G. (2010). Towards evidence-based, quality-controlled health promotion: the Dutch recognition system for health promotion interventions. *Health Education Research, 25,* 1100-1106.

Carey, M., Buchan, H., & Sanson-Fischer, R. (2009). The cycle of change: implementing best-evidence clinical practice. *International Journal for Quality in Health Care, 21*, 37–43.

Chorpita, B. F., Bernstein, A., & Daleiden, E. L. (2011). Empirically guided coordination of multiple evidence-based treatments: An illustration of relevance mapping in children's mental health services. *Journal of Consulting and Clinical Psychology, 79*, 470–480.

Chou, R. (2008a). Using evidence in pain practice. Part I: Assessing quality of systematic reviews and clinical practice guidelines. *Pain Medicine, 9,* 518-530.

Chou, R. (2008b). Using evidence in pain practice. Part II: Interpreting and applying systematic reviews and clinical practice guidelines. *Pain Medicine, 9,* 531-541.

Cook, B, G., Smith, G. J. & Tankersley, M. (2012). In K. R. Harris, S. Graham, and T. Urdan (Editors-in-Chief), *APA Educational Psychology Handbook: Vol. 1. Theories, Constructs, and Critical Issues* (pp. 495-527) San Diego,, CA: Academic Press.

Cooper, H. (2010). *Research Synthesis and Meta-Analysis: A Step-by-Step Approach* (4th Ed.). Thousand Oaks, CA: Sage.

Cooper, H., Hedges, L. V. & Valentine, J.C. (Eds.) (2009). *The Handbook of Research Synthesis and Meta-Analysis*. (2nd Ed.). New York: Russell Sage Foundation.

Drotar, D. (2010). Editorial: A call for replications of research in pediatric psychology and guidance for authors. *Journal of Pediatric Psychology, 35*, 801–805.

Dozois, D. J. (2013). Psychological treatments: Putting evidence into practice and practice into evidence. *Canadian Psychology, 54,* 1-11.

Evangelou, E., Ioannidis, J. P. A., & Patsopoulos, N. A. (2007). Uncertainty in heterogeneity estimates in meta-analyses. *BMJ: British Medical Journal, 335: 7626,* 914–916.

Farmington, D. P. (2006). Methodological quality and the evaluation of anti-crime programs. *Journal of Experimental Criminology, 2*, 329-337.

Fingeld-Connett, D. (2010). Generalizability and transferability of metasynthesis research findings. *Journal of Advanced Nursing, 66*, 246–254.

Hemsley-Brown, J., & Sharp, C. (2003). The use of research to improve professional practice: A systematic review of the literature. *Oxford Review of Education, 29,* 449-470.

Imbens, G. W. & Lemieux, T. (2008). Regression discontinuity designs: A guide to practice. *Journal of Econometrics, 142,* 615-635.

Jenson, W, A., Clark, E., Kircher, J. C., & Kristjansson, S. D. (2007). Statistical reform: Evidence-based practice, meta-analyses, and single subject designs. *Psychology in the Schools, 44,* 483-493.

Jitendra, A. K., Burgess, C. & Shigajria, M. (2011). Cognitive strategy instruction for improving expository text comprehension of students with learning disabilities: The quality of evidence. *Exceptional Children, 77,* 135-159.

Jüni, P., Witshci, A., Bloch, R., & Egger, M. (1999). The hazards of scoring the quality of clinical trials for meta-analysis. *Journal of the American Medical Association, 282*, 1054-1060.

Linkov, I., Welle, P., Loney, D., Tkachuk, A., Canis, L., Kim, J. B. & Bridges, T. (2011). Use of multicriteria decision analysis to support weight of evidence evaluation. *Risk Analysis, 31,* 1211-1225.

Krainovich-Miller, B., Haber, J., & Jacobs, S. K. (2009). Evidence-based practice challenge: Teaching critical appraisal of systematic reviews and clinical practice guidelines to graduate students. *Journal of Nursing Education, 48,*186-195.

Miller, J., & Schwarz, W. (2011). Aggregate and individual replication probability within an explicit model of the research process. *Psychological Methods, 16*, 337–360.

Montague, M. & Dietz, S. (2009). Evaluating the evidence base for cognitive strategy instruction and mathematical problem solving. *Exceptional Children, 75,* 285-302.

National Registry of Evidence-Based Programs and Practices. (2007). *NREPP review criteria*. Retrieved April 26, 2009, from http://www.nrepp.samhsa.gov/review-quality.asp.

Odom, S. L., Brantlinger, E., Gersten, R., Horner, R. H., Thompson, B. & Harris, K. R. (2005). Research in special education: Scientific methods and evidence-based practices. *Exceptional Children, 71,* 137-148.

Rubin, A., & Parrish, D. (2007). Problematic phrases in the conclusions of published outcome studies: Implications for evidence-based practice. *Research on Social Work Practice, 17*, 334-347.

Schalock, R. L., Verdugo, M. A., & Gomez, L. E. (2011). Evidence-based practices in the field of intellectual and developmental disabilities: An international consensus approach. *Evaluation and Program Planning, 34,* 273-282.

Schneider, B., Carnoy, M., Kilpatrick, J., Schmidt, W. H., & Shavelson, R. J. (2007). *Estimating causal effects using experimental and observational designs* (report from the Governing Board of the American Educational Research Association Grants Program). Washington, DC: American Educational Research Association.

Schraw, G. & Patell, E. (2013). Using principles of evidence-based practice to improve prescriptive recommendations. *Educational Psychology Review, 25,* 345-351.

Shadish, W. R. (1995). The logic of generalization: Five principles common to experiments and ethnographies. *American Journal of Community Psychology, 23*, 419-428.

Shadish, W. R., Cook, T. D., & Campbell, D. T. (2002). *Experimental and Quasi-Experimental Designs for Generalized Causal Inference.* Boston, MA: Houghton Mifflin.

Sherman, L. W., & Gottfredson, D. (1997). Appendix: Research methods. In L. Sherman, D. Gottfredson, D. MacKenzie, J. Eck, P. Reuter, & S. Bushway, *Preventing crime: What works, what doesn't, what's promising: A report to the United States Congress.* Washington, DC: U.S. Office of Justice Programs.

Smith, S. W., Daunic, A. P. & Taylor, G. G. (2007). Treatment fidelity in applied educational research: Expanding the adoption and application of measures to ensure evidence-based practice. Education and Treatment of Children, 30, 121-134.

Slavin, R. E. (2008). What works? Issues in synthesizing educational program evaluations. *Educational Researcher, 37,* 5-14.

Staines, G. L. (2008). The causal generalization paradox: The case of treatment outcome research. *Review of General Psychology, 12*, 236–252.

Valentine, J. C., & Cooper, H. (2008). A systematic and transparent approach for assessing the methodological quality of intervention effectiveness research: The Study Design and Implementation Assessment Device (Study DIAD). *Psychological Methods, 13*, 130-149.

Wecker, C. (2013). How to support prescriptive statements by empirical research: Some missing parts. *Educational Psychology Review, 25,* 1-18.

Westen, D. & Bradley, R. (2005). Empirically supported complexity: Rethinking evidence-based practice in psychotherapy. *Current Directions in Psychological Science, 14,* 266-271.

What Works Clearinghouse . (2008) . *What Works Clearinghouse procedures and standards handbook(Version 2.0)* . Washington , DC : Institute of Education Sciences, U.S. Department of Education . Retrieved from http://ies.ed.gov/ncee/wwc/references/idocviewer/doc.aspx?docid=19&tocid=1

Wilczynski, S. M. (2012). Risk and strategic decision-making in developing evidence-based practice guidelines. *Education and Treatment of Children, 35,* 291-311.

In: Evidence-Based Medicine and Practices
Editor: Ross T. Barnett
ISBN: 978-1-63482-362-3

Chapter III

Leadership, Ethics, and the Adoption of Evidence Based Medicine among Leaders of Internal Medicine and Surgery

Ronald Bogdasarian*[*]*, BA
The Commonwealth Medical College, Scranton, PA, US

Abstract

Background: Leadership, ethics and the adoption of evidence-based medicine (EBM) are interrelated components of modern medical care. In today's medical world, cost-effectiveness, patient safety and outcomes are paramount. EBM is at the forefront while engrained medical traditions are scrutinized at an increasing rate. This shift in paradigm requires strong leadership. With this complicated arrangement, exploration and comparison of the concepts of leadership, ethics, and EBM in two prominent areas of healthcare, general internal medicine and surgery, is a valuable exercise.

[*] E-mail: RBogdasarian@tcmc.edu.

Objective: The primary objective of this work is to review the literature on leadership and ethics in the field of internal medicine compared to surgery and examine how they affect the adoption of EBM. The secondary objective is to identify aspects of leadership, ethics, and the implementation of EBM within internal medicine and surgery that may serve to improve the other discipline.

Design: A review of the literature using Pubmed and Embase was performed. Keywords included leadership in internal medicine, leadership in surgery, ethics in internal medicine, ethics in surgery, evidence-based medicine in internal medicine, and evidence-based medicine in surgery.

Setting: The Commonwealth Medical College, Scranton, PA.

Results/Conclusion: The study identifies multiple similar qualities of leadership in internal medicine and surgery, especially the broad use of transformational leadership. While the less tangible qualities of charisma and personality are recognized, leaders who are willing to educate colleagues and work to solve problems with the healthcare system are required to generate acceptance of EBM by a healthcare team. Differences in leadership style that might affect the adoption of EBM exist between internal medicine and surgery. Internal medicine depends more on the culture of the team, while surgery depends more on the influence of powerful individual leaders. Other differences included internal medicine's greater appreciation for patient participation in care while surgical leaders are acknowledged most for technical skill and the ability to teach. Notably, both internal medicine and surgery ethical leaders refrain from conflicts of interest, especially regarding the increasing financial responsibilities, in order to maintain personal morals and the trust and respect of their healthcare teams. Ethical leaders in internal medicine place the patient's autonomy above the decisions of the medical team. Ethical leaders in surgery make appropriate decisions regarding heroic and end-of-life care. There are inherent differences between internal medicine and surgery that challenge the cross-over of leadership qualities from one discipline to the other. However, the differences in leadership style that do exist provide potential areas of improvement for each.

Keywords: leadership, medicine, surgery, ethics, evidence based

Background

In this review of the literature we explore the differences between internal medicine and surgery with regard to leadership and leadership's interface with ethics and the adoption of evidence-based medicine (EBM). We examine our findings and search for lessons that may benefit the art and practice of each discipline, particularly regarding the adoption of EBM. Today, a large portion of the leadership in healthcare is derived from non-physician, organizational management. This chapter will focus on physician leadership and ethics and their roles in the adoption of EBM.

A large body of literature describes two major systems of leadership—transformational and transactional leadership. Transformational leadership results in an environment in which team members feel personally connected to the goal. This system is often utilized in situations requiring broad change [1]. Transactional leadership is suited for use in emergency situations in which grand change is not necessary. It relies on rewards and punishments [2].

Much of the literature on leadership in medicine and surgery focuses on the team and a stepwise process, conforming more with the transformational system [3, 4, 5].

First, the leader, utilizing qualities such as charisma, confidence, wisdom, and inspirational communication, instills a common goal and culture within the team [6].

Second, while an active member of the clinical team, the physician leader is an excellent delegator and ensures that all members feel comfortable and important.

Third, the leader properly assesses performance and ensures completion of tasks.

Fourth, he or she constantly reflects in order to improve performance. These are the basics of medical leadership and are generally shared by internal medicine and surgery leaders. How, though, do leaders of medicine and surgery differ? Can these qualities cross over to improve leadership in the opposite discipline, and can these improvements lead to better implementation of EBM?

Strong ethics are essential for proper healthcare and leadership. Physicians are often presented with challenging ethical dilemmas which require familiarity with the fundaments of ethics. Both internal medicine and surgery leaders have a strong grasp on the principles of autonomy, beneficence, nonmaleficence, justice, the intricacies of informed consent, durable power of attorney and healthcare proxies [7, 8]. Are there other emphasized areas of ethics in healthcare today? How do ethics, cost-effective medicine, and EBM interrelate in the practice of healthcare leaders?

Today, EBM has a permanent place in medical practice and increasingly directs medical care. Many healthcare practitioners lament the loss of control over their abilities to make their own healthcare decisions. For this reason, knowledge of physician leadership and how it differs between internal medicine and surgery should prove valuable to improve the art and practice of medicine, healthcare professional satisfaction and patient outcomes.

Materials and Methods

Pubmed and Embase were used to review the literature. Keywords included leadership in internal medicine, leadership in surgery, ethics in internal medicine, ethics in surgery, evidence-based medicine in internal medicine and evidence-based medicine in surgery.

Results

Leadership in Internal Medicine

In addition to the transformational stepwise process of goal oriented leadership within the team environment, the literature presents multiple qualities of the strong internal medicine leader. Heavily emphasized is acceptance of change which has clear implications for the adoption of EBM over non-evidence supported traditional practices [9, 10, 11].

Further highlighted is teamwork, especially in interdisciplinary teams with emphasis on the patient as a team member [12, 13]. Two 2014 articles from the *Journal of General Internal Medicine* state that internal medicine leaders are inspired by their patients [14, 15]. Another 2014 article from the *Journal of General Internal Medicine* indicates that shared decision-making by the physician and patient, when evidence-based options and uncertainty are discussed, can lead to improved patient satisfaction [16].

A 2007 article from the *American Journal of Medical Quality* asserted that great internal medicine leaders direct attention to problems with the system, rather than with individual employees when an error causes harm to a patient [17]. This indicates that when a leader is dissatisfied with the implementation of EBM by a co-worker, he or she should examine the system in place meant to ensure the proper practice of EBM. This re-evaluation of the system, rather than a reprimand of a single employee or colleague, may help to improve the overall adoption of EBM.

Ethics in Internal Medicine

The literature expands upon the basic ethical principles mentioned in the background section. In a world where clinical leaders are becoming members of administration, conflict of interest and issues regarding financial honesty and fraud are paramount for the ethical leaders of internal medicine [18, 19, 20]. A 2013 article from the *Journal of Taibah Univiversity of Medical Science* notes multiple qualities of the internal medicine ethical leader, including "altruism, accountability, excellence, duty, honor and integrity, and respect for others." These leaders resist "abuse of power, sexual harassment, conflicts of interest, professional arrogance, physician impairment, and fraud in research" [21].

In order to accomplish the implementation of EBM through transformational leadership, in which a healthcare team becomes personally connected to the goal, the leader in internal medicine must be ethically sound. Conflicts of interest and fraud in research may undermine a healthcare team's trust in the evidence behind EBM and lead to reduced acceptance of new medical practices.

As explained previously, including the patient in decision making leads to increased patient satisfaction. Including the patient as an active member of the team was considered to be ethically essential for the internal medicine leader [14, 15]. Likewise, transparency and honestly with patients are also indispensable qualities of the internal medicine ethical leader [22].

Evidence Based Medicine in Internal Medicine

Much of the literature agrees that, in order for an internal medicine team to accept EBM, a culture of acceptance of change is paramount. This culture of change, resulting in the adoption of evidence-based practices, occurs in locations with strong hierarchal leadership and strong opinion leaders [23, 24]. These leaders are often seniors with time to reflect and learn. In other words, in order to be a leader, one cannot be overwhelmed by the daily routine to the point wheresuch that he or she cannot engage in novel medical learning [25]. These individuals must also be willing to "do what it takes to remove obstacles" to quality improvement such as poorly supported traditional beliefs and approaches. These leaders must be willing to take the time to share information and new knowledge on EBM and do so in a clear, concise manner [26].

Leadership in Surgery

Much of the literature on leadership in surgery states that confidence and speed pertaining to technical skill is essential for the leader in surgery [27, 28]. A surgeon who proves the worth of EBM through his or her own practice is more likely to convince others to train using similar practices.

The abilities to teach and mentor are highly regarded qualities of the surgical leader. A 2013 paper from the *International Journal of Surgery* takes this a step further, explicitly differentiating surgery from internal medicine. The authors comment that great surgical leaders take routine processes, such as check lists, and transform them into rich learning experiences [29]. In surgery, leaders who are able to employ this strategy in their support of EBM should be more successful.

The literature also highlights the ability to communicate in a democratic fashion in order to accomplish tasks with those with different ideals, personalities, and even goals [30, 31]. A 2014 study from *Health Affairs* states that humility is a key trait of the most respected surgical leaders. These leaders, while maintaining goals, are able to accept failure and are willing to communicate and cooperate with others to correct errors [32, 33]. Surgical leaders are also respected for "incisive, imaginative, [and] innovative scientific minds" [34]. One 1997 article from *Acta Neurochirurgica* discusses at length the importance of awareness to one's surroundings, objectives, and problems [35]. Interestingly, a 2013 article from the *Canadian Journal of Surgery* discusses the importance of personal development, especially in personal health and exercise in surgical leaders [36]. While not as prominent in the literature as technical skill and the ability to teach, these additional qualities may add to the recognition of the surgical leader and his or her ability to engage co-workers in the adoption of EBM.

In a glimpse into the minds of what influences surgical residents, a paper from *Aesthetic Plastic Surgery* describes "informal leadership". This concept refers to respect that is earned through consistent success in difficult situations, and can only be bestowed by peers. This "informal leadership" is distinct from one's title, or "formal leadership", which can be acquired by a surgeon who does not possess innate leadership qualities [37]. Surgical residents often gravitate to these surgeons who describe personal anecdotes of exciting, heroic experiences. While some may argue that these anecdotal experiences are exciting because they inherently diverge from the common, algorithmic EBM, these leaders are in a position to reaffirm the importance of EBM in everyday practice.

Ethics in Surgery

As in internal medicine, the literature on ethics in surgery heavily recognizes the good leader's resistance to conflicts of interest [38, 39]. Leaders in surgery are becoming more involved in administration, the financial aspects of care, and funding for research. The literature indicates that leaders in surgery must also avoid unethical practices in order to maintain co-workers trust for the implementation of EBM. The literature on ethics in surgery also emphasizes the leader's ability to decide when heroic care is appropriate [40, 41]. End-of-life care and heroic care are often technically difficult, expensive, and controversial. An in depth discussion on the specifics of EBM in this area of medicine is beyond the scope of this chapter. However, surgeons who are experienced and are capable of making difficult medical decisions, while remaining sensitive to the families of patients, are in a strong position to lead the adoption of EBM in this area.

Evidence Based Medicine in Surgery

Much literature focuses on the surgical leader's acceptance of EBM, which indicates that there is greater resistance to change and the adoption of EBM in surgery than in internal medicine, at least regarding engrained, everyday practices [42]. Again, the ability to teach is one of the most highly regarded qualities of leaders in surgery and is essential for theto propagation ofing evidence-based practices. The literature emphasized the open-mindedness of surgical opinion leaders who are called upon to accept EBM and show expertise and technical skill in its delivery. The literature suggests that opinion leaders are the driving force in a hierarchical system that is the structure in which attending and resident surgeons continue to learn. Thus, highly respected local opinion leaders as advocates for EBM is of utmost importance in surgery [43, 44, 45].

Discussion

As discussed in the background, the key components of leadership and ethics and their connection to the adoption of EBM are similar between internal medicine and surgery. There are, however, many notable differences.

Leadership

The literature indicatessuggests that leaders of both internal medicine and surgery tend to utilize a transformational, structured approach. Leaders generate a clear goal that members of the team identify with which supports a culture of agreement and productivity. Leaders put team members in positions to succeed and feel important. Leaders evaluate success as the team progresses. Once a goal is achieved, leaders reflect in order to improve for the future. This transformational method of leadership is well suited for the movement towards the EBM model.

Differences in leadership qualities between internal medicine and surgery include the following. Leaders of internal medicine accept the patient as a member of the team and are even "inspired" by their patients more often than their surgical counterparts. An essential quality of leadership in surgery is technical skill which can only be said for a small subset of internal medical physicians who perform a large volume of procedures [46]. Notably, the ability to teach is more commonly emphasized in the literature on surgical leaders than on internal medicine leaders.

These differences likely arise from the inherent differences between internal medicine and surgery. Internal medicine physicians traditionally spend more time conversing with patients in order to gather large volumes of information for management of multiple problems. These physicians receive praise as leaders for their ability to educate, comfort, and include patients in decision making. In surgery, much of the time spent with a patient is in the operating room where technical skill and outcomes are regarded as most important. While surgeons are still respected for good communication with patients, the emphasis is on the operative result. It is important to stress that discussions with patients should include education about evidence-based options for care. This results in the greatest patient satisfaction.

Due to the inherent differences between medicine and surgery, it is difficult to identify many areas of leadership that could cross over to the other discipline and improve the acceptance of EBM specifically. That said, possibilities areas for improvement include the following. In surgery, the technically savvy opinion leader has great potential for generating a more powerful culture change and should not be satisfied with simply providing an example of EBM to his or her peers. In internal medicine, while educating his or her colleagues and residents, the internal medicine leader should strive to create rich learning experiences from the repetitive daily routines that are part of EBM. Ultimately, all leaders should work to enhance the acknowledged strengths of their discipline's leadership style if they wish to increase the adoption of EBM.

Ethics

Many similarities exist regarding the ethics of internal medicine and surgery leaders. Both leaders have a strong grasp of the core principles of ethics, including autonomy, beneficence, nonmaleficence, justice, the proper use of informed consent, durable power of attorney and healthcare proxies.

Increasingly, both medical and surgical leaders are more involved in administration, finances, and funding for research. Recent literature focuses on the leader's refrainment from conflicts of interest that are possible in these positions. Internal medicine and surgery leaders must embrace this ethical pillar. Trust and respect from the healthcare team are necessary for change and the acceptance of EBM.

An important area of consideration regarding ethics is end-of-life care and heroic care. The literature indicates that internal medicine leaders focus more on the physician-patient relationship, while surgery leaders focus on when and when not to operate. While many surgical leaders do enjoy strong relationships with their patients during end-of-life care, the literature indicates that this is an area where surgeons could learn from their medical counterparts in order to strengthen this relationship. It is unclear, however, if this could enhance the adoption of EBM in surgery with regard to this area of healthcare. Alternatively, a focus on the willingness to make difficult decisions in end-of-life care is acknowledged as an important, albeit controversial, area in need of change toward EBM for both internal medicine and surgery leaders.

Evidence Based Medicine

The literature agrees that leaders in both internal medicine and surgery are at the forefront of the adoption of EBM. The manner in which EBM is encouraged differs, however.

The literature indicates that internal medicine leaders must create culture changes within their teams. Strong opinion leaders who are not overwhelmed by daily practice are required to generate these changes. Surgery is similar in that respected opinion leaders are essential, but there is less emphasis on culture change as a process.

The difference is subtle. Opinion leaders in internal medicine are important, but it is the cultural environment of the team that is most crucial. The literature indicates that surgery employs a powerful hierarchal system. In this system, the leaders have earned high regard due to their skills and ability to teach. These surgical leaders are able to influence the practice of their followers more so than the surgical culture does. As described previously, the surgical opinion leader may enjoy increased success in his followers' implementation of EBM if he works to generate culture change.

Conclusion

Most leaders in both internal medicine and surgery rely on the transformational form of leadership. The adoption of EBM by a team fits this leadership model well and is utilized by both groups of leaders. While the basics of leadership are similar, many of the differences between internal medicine and surgery leaders are due to the inherent differences in the respective disciplines. Even so, many leaders in each field bridge the gap and look to their colleagues in the other field for areas of potential improvement.

Key to the success of these physician and surgeon leaders is the sense of teamwork. They are confident and capable within their own realms of practice to the extent that they are able to diversify and enjoy aspects of the other group. While there are many specifics of leadership that can be improved upon by each group of leaders, such as patient centeredness for surgeons, teaching style, and technical skills for physicians and decisions regarding end-of-life care, it is most important to recall that physicians and surgeons are all members of the same team. All physicians and surgeons should share a common culture of teamwork so that colleagues may practice the most proven forms of medicine and patients may enjoy the best outcomes possible.

It is important to repeat that the material from this chapter comes from a literature review. The differences in leadership style, ethics and use of EBM between internal medicine and surgery were retrieved based on their relative presence in the literature. Although the literature may emphasize certain areas of leadership more in one discipline, this does not mean that leaders in the other discipline are not strong in that area.

Weaknesses of this review include the following. We did not differentiate among leadership in practice size or style or academic or community environment. We did not explore the topics of gender or race. We did not discuss non-physician leadership or the relationship between clinical leaders and administration. Healthcare costs, patient safety and outcomes are among the pre-eminent issues of healthcare today. The strongest of clinical leaders should have the ability to connect administrative leadership with the clinical work force in order to facilitate a relationship that benefits the three parties involved: the healthcare organization, clinicians, and patients. In this light, clinical leaders are more frequently assuming administrative rolls [47, 48]. In this review of the literature, the author attempted to withhold opinion.

Acknowledgments

I would like to acknowledge Bridget Conlogue of The Commonwealth Medical College Library for her vital contributions to this chapter.

We received no funding for the production of this work.

References

[1] Transformational leadership. Wikipedia. http://en.wikipedia.org/wiki/Transformational_leadership. Accessed 8/14/14.

[2] Transactional leadership. Wikipedia. http://en.wikipedia.org/wiki/Transactional_leadership. Accessed 8/14/14.

[3] Richard MJ, Bohmer MB, Ch, B. Leading Clinicians and Clinicians Leading. *N. Engl. J. Med.* 2013; 368:1468-1470. doi: 10.1056/NEJMp1301814.

[4] Duda, RB. Physician and scientist leadership in academic medicine: strategic planning for a successful academic leadership career. *Current Surg.* 2004; 61:175-177.

[5] Oza, SK, Miao, E, Pierce, R, Kuo, A, Van Schaik, S. Development of a leadership observation and feedback tool (LOFT). *Journ. of Gen. Intern Med.* 2013; 28(1): 459.

[6] Dine CJ, Khan JM, Abella BS, Asch DA, Shea JA. Key elements of clinical physician leadership at an academic medical center. *Journ. Grad. Med. Edu.* 2011; 3(1): 31–36. doi: 10.4300/JGME-D-10-00017.1.

[7] Ethical Decision Making in Obstetrics and Gynecology*. ACOG Committee Opinion no. 390. American College of Obstetricians and Gynecologists. *Obstet. Gynecol* 2007;110:1479-87.

[8] Mayer DM, Nurmohamed S, Trevino LK, Shapiro DL, Schminke M. Encouraging employees to report unethical conduct internally: it takes a village. *Org. Behav. and Hum. Decis Proc*. 2013; 89-103.

[9] Williams BC, Fisseha S, Williams J, Mullan P. Educating for change: Medical students develop organizational leadership skills through student-driven community based field projects. *Journ of Gen Intern Med*. 2014; 29(1): 516-517.

[10] Paryizi N, Shahaney S, Martin G, Ahmad A, Moghu M l. Instigating change: trainee doctors' perspective. *Postgrad Med. J*. 2013; 89:572-577. doi:10.1136/postgradmedj-2011-000370rep.

[11] Ball M, Lindberg D, Masic I. Special Tribute on Morris F. Collen: Charismatic leader of medical informatics. *Acta Inform Med*. 2014; 22(1): 4-5. doi:10.5455/aim.2014.22.4-5

[12] Rose SA, Jackson N, Fenner BP, Capel B, Rudy D. Promoting positive change in the residency experience through discovery of resident values. *Journ of Gen. Intern Med*. 2014; 185-186.

[13] Kim CS, King E, Stein J, Robinson E, Salameh M, O'Leary KJ. Unit-based interprofessional leadership models in six US hospitals. *J. Hosp. Med*. 2014; 9(8):545-50. doi: 10.1002/jhm.2200.

[14] Jackson N, Fenner B, Capel BJ, Rudy D. Promoting positive change in the residency experience through discovery of resident values. *Journ. of Gen. Intern Med*. 2014; 62(2): 582.

[15] Radhakrishnan P, Thorn P. Story telling: my most memorable patient – lessons in humanism, reflection, and the development of expertise. *Journ. of Gen. Intern Med*. 2014; 29(1): 534.

[16] Berger Z. Navigating the unknown: shared decision-making in the face of uncertainty. *Journ of Gen. Intern Med*. 2014: In press,

[17] Clarke JR, Lerner JC, Marella W. The role for leaders of healthcare organizations in patient safety. *Am. J. Med. Qual*. 2007; 22: 311-318.

[18] Pisano ED, Golden RN, Schweitzer L. Conflict of interest policies for academic health system leaders who work with outside corporations. *JAMA*. 2014; 311(11): 1111-1112. doi:10.1001/jama.2014.788.

[19] Campbell C, Wolf D, Hoover N, Rees T, Smith S. Incomplete conflict of interest (COI) disclosures-analysis of recent publications. *Cur. Med. Resear and Opin*. 2013; 29(1): 9-19. doi:10.1185/03007995.2013.780866.

[20] DeCamp M, Farber NJ, Torke AM, George M, Berger Z, Keirns CC, Kaldjian LC. Ethical challenges for accountable care organizations: a structured review. *J. Gen. Intern Med*. 2014. Ahead of Press.

[21] Kasule OH. Medical professionalism and professional organizations. *Journ Taibah Univ. Med. Sci.* 2013; 8(3): 137–141. doi: 10.1016/j.jtumed.2013.09.003.

[22] Chervenak FA, McCullough LB. An ethical framework for identifying, preventing, and managing conflicts confronting leaders of academic health centers. *Aca Med.* 2004; 79(11):1056-61.

[23] Shahzad S, Zareen H. Perception of leadership among health managers working in tertiary level hospitals. *Journ Ayub. Med. Coll.* 2012; 24(1): 96-100.

[24] Curran GM, Thrush CR, Smith JL, Owen RR, Ritchie M, Chadwick D. Implementing research findings into practice using clinical opinion leaders: barriers and lessons learned. *Jt Comm J. Qual Patient Saf.* 2005; 31(12):700-7.

[25] Swennen MHJ, Van Der Heijden GJ, Blijham GH, Kalkman CJ. Career stage and work setting create different barriers for evidence-based medicine. *J. Eval. Clin. Pract.* 2011; 17(4): 775-85.

[26] Davidow SL. Physicians taking the lead to improve patient care. *Jt Comm J. Qual. Improv.* 1999; 25(3):145-52.

[27] Briggs A, Raja AS, Joyce MF, Yule SJ, Jian W, Lipsitz SR, Havens JM. The impact of trauma team training on team leaders' non-technical skills during simulated trauma scenarios. *J. Surg. Res.* 2014; 186(2): 671-672. doi:10.1016/j.jss.2013.11.747.

[28] Jernigan AM, Stephens JP, Knight J. Surgeons as active leaders in the operating room: potential cost-saving behaviors. *Gynecologic Oncology.* 2014; 133(1): 35. doi:10.1016/j.ygyno.2014.03.107.

[29] Suliman A, Klaber RE, Warren OJ. Exploiting opportunities for leadership development of surgeons within the operating theatre. *Int. J. Surg.* 2013; 11(1): 6-11. doi: 10.1016/j.ijsu.2012.11.002.

[30] Robinson M, Macneily A, Afshar K, McInnes C, Lennox P, Carr N, Skarlicki D, Masterson J, Arneja J. Leadership in Canadian urology: what is the right stuff? *J. Surg. Edu.* 2013; 70(5): 606-612. doi: 10.1016/j.jsurg.2013.04.013.

[31] Souba WW. New ways of understanding and accomplishing leadership in academic medicine. *J. Surg. Res.* 2004; 117(2):177-86.

[32] Mello MM, Senecal SK, Kuznetsov Y, Cohn JS. Implementing hospital-based communication-and-resolution programs: lessons learned in New York City. *Health Aff.* 2014; 33(1): 30-38. doi: 10.1377/hlthaff.2013.0849.

[33] Hu Y, Parker SH, Arriaga AF, Peyre SE, Corso KA, Roth EM, Yule SJ, Greenberg CC. Follow the leader? The impact of leadership style on team performance in the OR. *J. Surg. Res.* 2013; 179(2).

[34] Shields CB. Leadership in neurosurgery. *Neurosurg.* 1989; 25(1): 1-5.

[35] Brock M. Leadership qualities in prominent neurosurgeons. *Acta Neurochir Suppl.* 1997; 69: 8-11.

[36] Klein G, Hussain N, Sprague S, Mehlman CT, Dogbey G, Bhandari M. Characteristics of highly successful orthopedic surgeons: a survey of orthopedic chairs and editors. *Can J. Surg.* 2013; 56(3):192–198. doi: 10.1503/cjs.017511.

[37] Prado A, Parada F. Leadership in plastic surgery today. *Aesthet Plas Surg.* 2010; 1-3.

[38] Minter RM, Angelos P, Coimbra R, Dale P, De Vera ME, Hardacre J, Hawkins W, Kirkwood K, Matthews JB, McLoughlin J, Peralta E, Schmidt M, Zhou W, Schwarze ML. Ethical management of conflict of interest: proposed standards for academic surgical societies. *J. Am. Coll. Surg.* 2011; 213(5): 677-82. doi: 10.1016/j.jamcollsurg.2011.08.003.

[39] Elliot BM. Conflict of interest and the society for vascular surgery. *J. Vasc. Surg.* 2011; 54(3): 3-11.

[40] Roberts DJ, Zygun DA, Kirkpatrick AW, Ball CG, Faris PD, Bobrovitz N, Robertson HL, Stelfox HT. A protocol for a scoping and qualitative study to identify and evaluate indications for damage control surgery and damage control interventions in civilian trauma patients. *BMJ Open.* 2014; 4(7): doi:10.1136/bmjopen-2014-005634.

[41] Civetta JM. Critical care: how should we evaluate our progress? *Crit Care Med.* 1992; 20(12): 1714-20.

[42] Escobar MA, McCullough LB. Responsibly managing ethical challenges of residency training: a guide for surgery residents, educators, and residency program directors. *J. Am. Coll. Surg.* 2006; 202: 531-535.

[43] Callahan CD, Adair D, Bozic KJ, Manning BT, Saleh JK, Saleh KJ. Orthopaedic surgery under national health reform: an analysis of power, process, adaptation, and leadership: AOA critical issues. *J. Bone Joint Surg. Am.* 2014; 96(13): 111.

[44] Stijntjes F, Obertop H. Evidence-based surgery. *Nederland Tijdschrift voor Geneeskunde.* 2008; 152(38): 2065-70.

[45] Young JM, Hollands MJ, Ward J, Holman CD. Role for opinion leaders in promoting evidence-based surgery. *Arch. Surg.* 2003; 138(7): 785-91.

[46] Chonde M, Intaphan J, Killu C. ACLS leadership training in medical residents and its effect on confidence. *Critic Care Med.* 2013; 41(12): 128-129.

[47] Mostashari F, Sanghavi D, McClellan M. Health Reform and Physician-Led Accountable Care: The Paradox of Primary Care Physician Leadership. *JAMA.* 2014; 311(18):1855-1856. doi:10.1001/jama.2014.4086.

[48] Satiani B, Sena J, Ruberg R, Ellison EC. Talent management and physician leadership training is essential for preparing tomorrow's physician leaders. *J. Vasc. Surg.* 2014; 59(2): 542-6. doi: 10.1016/j.jvs.2013.10.074.

In: Evidence-Based Medicine and Practices
Editor: Ross T. Barnett ISBN: 978-1-63482-362-3

Chapter IV

Comparative Analysis of Cost-Benefit and Cost-Effectiveness of All Types of Evidence-Based Medicine for All Clinical Conditions – QALY, HALY and Survival

Søren Ventegodt*
Quality of Life Research Center, Copenhagen, Denmark;
Research Clinic for Holistic Medicine and Nordic
School of Holistic Medicine, Copenhagen, Denmark;
Nordic School of Holistic Medicine, Copenhagen, Denmark;
Scandinavian Foundation for Holistic Medicine, Sandvika, Norway;
Interuniversity College, Graz, Austria

* Corresponding author: Søren Ventegodt, MD, MMedSci, EU-MSc-CAM, Director, Quality of Life Research Center, Frederiksberg Allé 13A,2.t.v., DK-1820 Copenhagen V, Denmark. Tel: +45-33-141113; E-mail: ventegodt@livskvalitet.org Website: www.livskvalitet.org.

Abstract

Aim: To compare cost-benefit and cost-effectiveness of all types of evidences-based medicine, both pharmaceuticals and non-drug CAM for all clinical conditions.

Method: Calculating therapeutic value ($TV=NNH_{total}/NNT$) and cost per cured patient (year 1-50) for 10 different types of evidence-based medicine. Cost is presented as EURO per cured patient, EURO per QALY, EURO per HALY, and number of harmed and killed patients per cured patient. The cost of one year of treatment was set to 2,000€, and the difference between healthy and sick to 20% (quality of life, self-rated health). *Results*: We found the most effective CAM-types(mind-body medicine, holistic medicine, shamanism) to be 100 times as cost-effective and 10.000 times less harmful compared to pharmaceuticals. The 50 years estimated cost for one patient cured was for: drugs 1,000,000€; physical therapy 100,000€; psychotherapy 100,000€; mind-body medicine 50,000€; holistic mind-body medicine 20,000€; one-session shamanistic healing with hallucinogenic drugs 2,000€. CAM is more efficient than drugs and has no side effects and adverse events, whereas treatment with drugs always has adverse effects and events. Only chemical medicine has mortality as adverse effect. *Interpretation*: To be useful medicine must have significant Therapeutic value (good ratio of benefits to harm: $TV \geq 1$) and documented long term effect and safety. The shift from drugs to CAM would improve health and quality of life radically in society and reduce harm to patients and the cost of healthcare to a small fraction. Strict laws should be introduced immediately in all countries to stop the pharmaceutical industry from promoting drugs without Therapeutic value, and from repressing CAM.

Keywords: CAM, cost-efficacy, quality of life, holistic medicine, mind-body medicine, biomedicine, non-drug medicine, side effects, adverse effects, therapeutic value, evidence-based medicine, public health, law

Introduction

The US National Center for Complementary and Alternative Medicine (NCCAM) has suggested that all evidence-based medicine is categorized into six major categories: Biomedicine using drugs, and five major categories of complementary and alternative medicine (CAM). We have found it useful to expand this into a revised system of 10-classes of evidence-based medicine, that includes all medicine in general [1], as we agree to the viewpoint often presented in JAMA (Journal of the American Medical Association) that CAM and biomedicine must be one integrated medical system of evidence-based medicine [2] (see Table 1).

Table 1. Classification of medicine (including CAM and biomedicine) into 10 principal classes, Class 1 and 2 are chemical medicines; 3-10 are informational medicines

1. Chemical medicine (biomedicine with bioactive molecules)
2. Chemical CAM (flower medicine, herbal medicine, diets, minerals, vitamins etc.)
3. Body-medicine (Low-energy types: massage, reflexology, physical therapy, physiotherapy, spa, sauna etc; High-energy times: chiropractics etc.)
4. Mind-medicine (psychotherapy - psychodynamic, cognitive, gestalt etc.- psychoanalysis, meditation, no-touch sexology, couching, healing music)
5. Spirit-medicine (philosophical interventions, energy medicine, prayers, spiritual healing (i.e., Reichi), shamanism, spiritual CAM (i.e., crystal healing) etc.)
6. Mind-body medicine (acupuncture, acupressure, homeopathy, manual sexology, body-psychotherapy, Reichian bodywork, Rosen therapy, ergo therapy etc.)
7. Body-spirit medicine (prayer involving physical activity like in Tibetan Buddhist-style meditation, pilgrimage etc.)
8. Holistic body-mind-spirit medicine - including existential therapy (holistic medicine, clinical medicine, clinical holistic medicine, holistic body-psychotherapy, holistic bodywork, the sexological examination, holistic mind-body medicine, biodynamic body-psychotherapy, tantric bodywork and massage, holistic sexology, Native American rituals).
9. Chemical-body-mind-spirit medicine (shamanism with peyote, Ayuhuasca, magic mushrooms, Grof's LSD-psychotherapy etc.)
10. Social and environmental medicine (coaching, work-related personal development programs, stress management, leadership training, gardening, aesthetic architecture, FengShui etc.)

In this chapter we want to examine the cost-benefit and cost-efficiency of the 10 different types of evidence-based medicine. We want to look at the ration benefit-to-harm (often called therapeutic value, TV), the cost of the production of quality of life (QALY, or global QOL per EURO) and self-rated health (HALY) and the cost of health in patient damage and mortality.

Methods

Today there are four major population health measures permitting morbidity and mortality to be simultaneously evaluated: survival, QALYs (quality of life-adjusted life years), HALYs (health-adjusted life years) and DALYs (disability- adjusted life years). In this paper we will only estimate survival, QALYs and HALYs.

The method is estimating the general numbers from metaanalyses, preferably Cochrane reviews, and, when possible, meta-metaanalyses covering one or more of the different types of evidence-based medicine. We will include estimates from the leading medical journals of typical numbers of NNTs and NNHs. To make such a highest-level analysis where we look at all types of medicine for all clinical conditions we will need to simplify matters. When it comes to survival we regret to find the data in very bad condition as most studies do not include this extremely important measure; we therefore have given our best estimate based on the data available.

The prize of pharmaceutical drugs will be calculated from the Danish cost of drugs to more than two million chronic patients in Denmark using biomedicine; this number might be high compared to the number in developing countries were medicine often is sold cheaper. The prize of CAM treatments are also coming from Danish circumstances, where a year of therapy often is about 20 session costing around 2000€; in developing countries the prize is often a tenth of that. The calculation of QALY and HALY is using the knowledge on normal loss of quality of life and self-rated health when people get ill in Denmark; as we have a lot of social security to some extend compensating for loss of quality of life and health, the prize per QALY and HALY might be lower in less developed countries.

As our results are calculated based on estimate numbers we must admit have an uncertainty of +/- 100%, we believe our results to be correct within a factor three. As the differences between the different types of medicine are often a factor 10 or 100, this large uncertainty is still acceptable.

As the biggest problem in medical research today is bias from economical interests, we have avoided sources that might be strongly biased, like RCTs from pharmaceutical industry, overoptimistic estimates in reviews from CAM-journals not represented in MedLine/www.PubMed.gov etc.

Actually the process of limiting bias has been our biggest problem, forcing us to leaving out most of the sources often used in this type of analyses, like statistics made by public organs headed by people close to the pharmaceutical industry. Such statistics seems mostly to be extremely biased in favor of biomedicine.

There are many fundamental problems in biomedicine we could have addressed to make this study more thorough; there are problems from the practical use of drugs with low compliance, wrong diagnosis, errors in prescriptions and overmedication; there are problems with the RCTs at its very roots making the NNT and NNH numbers from industrial testing difficult to trust, and this paper is after all based on numbers coming from the pharmaceutical industries use of the RCT in testing its products. So we know that we are only scratching the surface of the problems in this paper.

We have wanted things to be so simple that complexity of things could not allow us to bias the paper our self; what happens in any complex procedure is that you unconsciously will take things in the direction you with or expect, and only by making things so simple that there are no steps to twist or manipulate can you truly avoid bias. We believe that the simplicity of our calculations and estimates has leaded us to trustworthy, fairly unbiased results.

Our main source of information is the Cochrane library. In former papers, where we have analyzed aspects of one of the 10 types of medicine, we have had several hundred references. In this paper we are using the whole Cochrane library as reference. To make the reference list of acceptable length we are only listing complementary material used in the study in the reference list.

Results

A. QALY and HALY

Based on the Cochrane library we have evaluated the benefit and harm from pharmaceutical drugs and the different CAM systems. We have looked at the likelihood to benefit using Number Needed to Treat (NNT), the likelihood to be harmed by the different adverse effects/side effects by using Number Needed to treat to Harm (NNH), and the total likelihood to get one side effect/adverse reaction or adverse event (NNH_{total}) and from this we have calculated the ratio "benefit to harm" called the Therapeutic value of the treatment ($TV=NNH_{total}/NNT$) [3, 4, 5], for the 10 different types of medicine, see Table 2.

While it for a long time, thanks to the many Cochrane reviews, has been easy to find NNT and NNH numbers for most pharmaceutical drugs (although there is almost no data on mortality caused by the drugs in spite of the fact that they are known to be very toxic), it has been more difficult to establish NNT and NNH numbers for the many different types of holistic and alternative medicine (CAM), and the relative harm of non-drug medicine had to be estimated from the number of reported cases in the literature [6]. Recently more than hundred Cochrane reviews have been made on a large number of CAM-types for a large number of clinical conditions, and NCCAM, the US research center for CAM, has published a number of reports on five major categories of CAM, allowing us for a far better estimate of NNHs and NNTs [7, 8] (see Table 2). As an example NCCAM has evaluated the number of patients treated every year in the US with massage therapy (therapeutic touch) and the number of patients experiencing significant side effects from such treatments; NCCAM found that 20,000,000 adults and 700.000 children are treated every year with very few patients harmed [9], allowing us to estimate NNH>1,000,000 for massage and similar types of therapeutic touch. Of the 145 Cochrane reviews of CAM analyzed by "Committee on the Use of Complementary and Alternative Medicine by the American Public" [8] 38,4% of the reviews showed a positive or possibly positive (12.4%) effect. These Cochrane reviews documented typical NNTs of 2-30, depending on CAM type, and typical NNHs of 1000-1.000.000. Typical NNTs and NNHs for the 10 types of evidence-based medicine are presented in table 2 [3, 5].

Two things are especially interesting for patient: 1) How efficient is the medicine? This is best known from Number Needed to Treat (NNT) telling how likely it is that the patient will benefit from the treatment. 2) How harmful is the medicine. The absolute harm is important but even more important is the ratio benefit to harm. Many patients will feel that a treatment is of therapeutic value if its advantages (statistically) dominate its disadvantages. The ratio benefit to harm is simplest expressed by the ratio $TV=NNH_{total}/NNT$, where NNTtotal is the total likelihood of getting a side/adverse effect or adverse event. Typical values of HHN_{total} and TV can also be found in Table 2.

In general chemical medicine, whether biomedical drugs or CAM (herbs, aromatic oils, diet changes etc.) have high NNH_{total}s and low TVs. The effect of chemical CAM seems to be less than pharmaceutical drugs, but it is a lot safer.

If you manipulate the biological informational system of the patient (for the scientific concept of biological information, see 12) instead of body chemistry, you seem to avoid side/adverse effects and adverse events. Some types of CAM has a low efficacy, but still the TV is high because of the relative safeness.

Table 2. Typical numbers for effect and harm, and the ration of *benefit to harm* for 10 classes of evidence-based medicine (NNTs, NNHs, NNH_{total}s and TVs)

CAM class	Short term effect (0-6 month)	Long term effect (6-24 month)	Side effects/adverse events	Total risk of harm	Therapeutic Value TV=NNH_{total}/NNT
	NNT	NNT	NNH	NNH_{total}	TV(6-24 month)
Class 1-Biomedicine (pharmaceuticals)	20 (5-50)	50 (5-100)	1-5	1-3	1-0.01
Class 2-CAM (Chemical CAM)	≥20	≥50	25 (allergy)	25	0.5
Class 3a-CAM (Physical therapy, low-energy i.e., massage, therapeutic touch)	2-4	6	>1.000.000	>1.000.000	167.000
Class 3b-CAM (Physical therapy, high-energy i.e. chiropractic treatment)	2-4	6	1000 (fractures)	1000	167
Class 4-CAM (Psychotherapy)*	3	6	>1.000.000	>1.000.000	167.000
Class 5-CAM (Spiritual therapy)	>10	>20	>1.000.000	>1.000.000	50.000
Class 6-CAM (Mind-Body medicine)	2	4	>1.000.000	>1.000.000	250.000
Class 7-CAM (Body-Spirit medicine)	Not known	Not known	>1.000.000	>1.000.000	Not known
Class 8-CAM (Holistic mind-body medicine)	2	1-2**	>1.000.000	>1.000.000	500.000-1.000.000
Class 9-CAM (Shamanism w. drugs etc.)***	1	1	>1000	>1000	>1000
Class 10-CAM (Social medicine)	1	10	>1.000.000	>1.000.000	100.000

Estimated from Cochrane reviews of RCTs and from clinical studies with chronic patients [3, 4, 5, 6, 8, 9, 10], see text.

*Some types of psychotherapy have short-term NNTs of 2-3 (STPP) and long term NNTs of 1-2 (LTPP) for mental, somatic and sexual health problems [see 3, 10]. **The effect of clinical holistic medicine and similar medical systems seem to continue to increase though time [11]. NNT: Number Needed to Treat. NNH: Number Needed to Harm, NNH_{total}: Total likelihood of getting one side effect/adverse effect or adverse event. TV: Therapeutic value, which here means ratio of benefit to harm. For a treatment to be of true value to patients, is must be efficient, with a low NNT number, and a high TV-number. ***Adverse effects, mostly brief reactive psychoses, are only seen with mentally ill patients [6].

Some types of CAM are both efficient and safe. Holistic mind-body medicine seems to be as safe as other kinds of CAM but more efficient and there has the highest TV. Interestingly, there are adverse effects of the drugs traditionally used in shamanism [6], giving shamanistic medicine the lowest TV of all CAM treatments; but if you look at the cost during a 50 years life span, Shamanism ends up looking the best of all known treatments (see table 6). As we do not want to return to Shamanism, we would like to give our tribute to the pre-modern medicine. Indigenous people often know much about medicine.

The cost of different drugs and different CAM treatment varies a great deal. Within every class of evidence-based medicine there are expensive and cheap alternatives. We have found I fair to set both a pharmaceutical and a CAM treatment to 2000€ per year, knowing that praying is cheaper and cancer-chemotherapy is more expensive. If you know the NNT-number and the cost of one patient treated, you can find the cost for one patient cured (or at least treated successfully) by multiplying these numbers (Cost of one patient cured = NNT x yearly treatment cost) (Table 3). The next year the cured patients will not cost anything but the patient not cured will still cost the yearly treatment cost. In this way can we estimate the 10 and 50 years cost of one patient cured (see table 3). If the NNT is very high, very few patients get cured and most become chronic patient. This is the case for pharmaceutical drugs so here the calculation is simple: The cost as times goes by is calculated as *yearly cost X time*. If all or most patients are cure in one or a few years, the calculation is similar simple: The total treatment cost is the one year treatment cost. When patients get better little by little, as in psychotherapy, a more complicated estimate must be made, accounting for the current recovery of patients. Our estimates of all ten classes are found in table 3. Due to lack of data we could not make estimates for Class 5 and 7.

If there are many adverse effects and events these cost sick-days, hospitalization etc. We know that drugs are always poisonous to some extent, and that it is estimated that there are now100,000 deaths a year in US hospitals directly caused by pharmaceuticaldrugs [13]. This is a huge cost but we have only included the direct cost to the drugs in our estimate. The true cost is likely to be several times larger.

A popular effect measure is QALY, or Quality Adjusted Life Years. The idea is simple: Survival has in itself no value; if you survive but suffer to en extreme extent it might be better if the doctor had not saved you in the first place. The secure that the patient gets value for money, the cost per QALY must be calculated. As QOL of life in general is 20% lower for ill people than for healthy [14] we can make a simple estimate of cost/QALY, presented in table 4.

The principles of the estimate are simple: If a patient is cured right away and stays healthy, and would have become a chronic patient without treatment, the cost for one cured patient is multiplied with the time the patient's health is improved. As very few patients are cured with biomedicine, the cost of one QALY becomes astronomic as the treatment continues for life without results – which is normally the case in Denmark where we have socialized biomedicine, free or very cheap for all chronic patients.

Table 3. Accumulated cost (number of patient with side effects/adverse effects and adverse events) for one patient cured through time (year one, ten and fifty) for 10 classes of evidence-based medicine

Continuous treatment (only stopped if the patients gets cured)	Cost per patient-year	Accumulated cost (€)		
	Per treted patient	per cured patient	per cured patient	per cured patient
	First year	First year	Year 10	Year 50
Medicine with drugs (chemical medicine) Class 1 – Chemical medicine[1]	2,000	≥100,000	≥200,000	≥1,000,000
Class 2-CAM (Chemical CAM)	2,000	>100,000	>200,000	>1,000,000
Non-drug CAM (informational medicine)				
Class 3-CAM (Physical therapy)	2,000	12,000	60,000	100,000
Class 4-CAM (Psychotherapy)	2,000	12,000	60,000	100,000
Class 5-CAM (Spiritual therapy)	Not known	Not known	Not known	Not known
Class 6-CAM (Mind-Body medicine)	2,000	8,000	30,000	50,000
Class 7–Body-Spirit medicine				
Class 8-CAM (Holistic mind-body medicine)	2,000	5,000	10,000	20,000
Class 9-CAM (Shamanism w. drugs)	500	600	800	2,000
Class 10-CAM (Social/environm. medicine)	5.000	50.000	350.000	500.000

[1](cost of biomedical examination, hospitalization, and treatment of adverse effects and events not included) (estimated round numbers, see text).

On the other hand will a QALY-unit, with an efficient CAM cure, with normally has the extra plus that patients not only stays healthy but also improves health through time (as they have learned the basic principles for human development) as times go by be relatively cheaper.

For every past year the quality of life and health is already paid, as shown in Table 4. Interestingly one-session shamanistic healing is far the cheapest kind of medicine, presumably explaining its great popularity in almost all pre-modern cultures.

Table 4. Accumulated cost of one QALY (Quality of life-adjusted Life Year) through time (year one, ten and fifty) for 10 classes of evidence-based medicine

Continuous treatment (only stopped if the patients gets cured)	QOL improvement from treatment (%) if successful	Prize of one QALY calculated from NNT and accumulated cost (table 3)		
	Global QOL	per cured patient	per cured patient	per cured patient
		First year	Year 10	Year 50
Medicine with drugs (chemical medicine) Class 1 – Chemical medicine[1]	20%	500,000	≥1,000,000	≥5,000,000
Class 2-CAM (Chemical CAM)	20%	>500,000	>1,000,000	>5,000,000
Non-drug CAM (informational medicine)				
Class 3-CAM (Physical therapy)	20%	60,000	300,000	60,000
Class 4-CAM (Psychotherapy)	20%	60,000	300,000	60,000
Class 5-CAM (Spiritual therapy)	20%	Not known	Not known	Not known
Class 6-CAM (Mind-Body medicine)	20%	40,000	180,000	40,000
Class 7–CAM Body-Spirit medicine	20%	Not known	Not known	Not known
Class 8-CAM (Holistic mind-body medicine)	20%	25,000	50,000	10,000
Class 9-CAM (Shamanism w. drugs)	20%	3000	4000	800
Class 10-CAM (Social/environm. medicine)	20%	250.000	1,750.000	2,500.000

[1](cost of biomedical examination, hospitalization, and treatment of adverse effects and events not included) (estimated round numbers, see text).

In one-session healing you are normally taken unto a daylong journey of guided self-exploration where you come to understand how you make yourself ill by the way you life and look at things. It's thus a life-style and philosophy of life intervention. From a theoretical point of view it might actually work.

Instead of QALYs, WHO often recommend the use of HALYs (and DALYs), which is exactly the same, only with health (most often self-rated health) instead of quality of life.

We know that the strongest measure of health is self-rated health [15-18], and we also know that sick people experience there health very much the same way as they experience their quality of life [14] allowing us again to use a difference of 20% between healthy and ill people. This gives us table 5, showing that mind-body medicine gives lots of health for the money, while chemical medicine and social medicine does not.

The harm caused by the 10 different types of evidence-based medicine as times goes by has been estimated in table 6. Patients using biomedicine for years without being cured, as is normally the case, are accumulating the harmful adverse effects and events caused by the pharmaceutical drugs. Non-drug CAM does not cause significant harm. The hallucinogenic drugs have some rare, but significant adverse effects but as shamanistic medicine is often very efficient with result that last for life due to increase self-awareness and self-insight, the harm inflicted over a life-span becomes similar to the level of harm inflicted by the other CAM systems, indicating that we might be more open to the potential benefits of pre-modern medicine and drug-induced one session healing, like Grof's LSD therapy [19].

B. Mortality

While it is generally agreed that CAM is not causing dead, and no specific examination of mortality therefore is needed, the opposite is the case when chemical drugs are used as medicine.

The drugs that are selected as medicine have all the classical qualities of the very toxic or mortal drugs: They pass into the bodies most sensitive organs (i.e., passes the blood-brain barrier), they are difficult to degrade by the body as they often consist of compounds (like polycyclic aromatic rings) not known to the biological organism through evolution so that there are no specific catabolic pathways for them in the liver and other organs specialized to degrade toxic substances, and they are selected for high biological activity. In the chemical lab such drugs are always classified as the most toxic substances.

Table 5. Accumulated cost of one HALY (Quality of life-adjusted Life Year) through time (year one, ten and fifty) for 10 classes of evidence-based medicine

Continuous treatment (only stopped if the patients gets cured)	Health improvement from treatment (%) if successful	Prize of one HALY calculated from NNT and accumulated cost (table 3)		
	Self-rated health	per cured patient	per cured patient	per cured patient
		First year	Year 10	Year 50
Medicine with drugs Class 1 – Chemical medicine[1]	20%	500,000	≥1,000,000	≥5,000,000
Class 2-CAM (Chemical CAM)	20%	>500,000	>1,000,000	>5,000,000
Non-drug CAM				
Class 3-CAM (Physical therapy)	20%	60,000	300,000	60,000
Class 4-CAM (Psychotherapy)	20%	60,000	300,000	60,000
Class 5-CAM (Spiritual therapy)	20%	Not known	Not known	Not known
Class 6-CAM (Mind-Body medicine)	20%	40,000	180,000	40,000
Class 7–CAM Body-Spirit medicine	20%	Not known	Not known	Not known
Class 8-CAM (Holistic mind-body medicine)	20%	25,000	50,000	10,000
Class 9-CAM (Shamanism w. drugs)	20%	3000	4000	800
Class 10-CAM (Social/environm. medicine)	20%	250.000	1,750.000	2,500.000

[1](cost of biomedical examination, hospitalization, and treatment of adverse effects and events not included) (estimated round numbers, see text).

Table 6. Accumulated harm through time (year one, ten and fifty) for 10 classes of evidence-based medicine- prize for one patient cured

Continuous treatment (only stopped if the patient gets cured)	Number of patients harmed For one patient cured	Accumulated harm (number of patients harmed per patient cured)		
	Self-rated health	per cured patient	per cured patient	per cured patient
	NNH_{total}	First year	Year 10	Year 50
Medicine with drugs Class 1 – Chemical medicine	3	17	25	50
Class 2-CAM (Chemical CAM)	25	2	4	5
Non-drug CAM				
Class 3a-CAM (Physical therapy, Low E) Class 3b-CAM (Physical therapy, High E.)	1,000,000 1,000	0.000,01 0,002	0.000,1 0,01	0.001 0,1
Class 4-CAM (Psychotherapy)	1,000,000	0.000,01	0.000,1	0.001
Class 5-CAM (Spiritual therapy)	1,000,000	Not known	Not known	Not known
Class 6-CAM (Mind-Body medicine)	1,000,000	0.000,01	0.000,1	0.001
Class 7–CAM Body-Spirit medicine	1,000,000	Not known	Not known	Not known
Class 8-CAM (Holistic mind-body medicine)	1,000,000	0.000,01	0.000,1	0.001
Class 9-CAM (Shamanism w. drugs)	1,000	0.001	0.001	0.001
Class 10-CAM (Social/environm. medicine)	1,000,000	0.000,01	0.000,1	0.001

You would therefore expect that whenever such drugs are applied to human beings the risk of mortality would be carefully monitored, but surprisingly this is not so.

The pharmaceutical companies have often systematically done everything they can to avoid measuring mortality when a new drug is tested [23].

Death by increased suicide rate is almost never measured for the psychopharmacological drugs, in spite of the fact that it has been known for decades that the drugs induce suicide [23].

Given the data on survival and mortality is of extremely poor quality it might be helpful to compare them to the toxic effect known for the classes of drugs in general, and it is well known that in the doses used for medicine the drugs do cause death. Table 7 summarized the findings found by leading members of the Cochrane organization consisting of around 2000 medical doctors and researchers who intent to give evaluations of effect and adverse effects/side effects of all types of medicine published according to the Cochrane protocol in Cochrane reviews [23].

It is easy to see that only chemical medicine is causing death which makes it mandatory to use a non-drug medicine whenever available.

Discussion

For a society the most important thing is to choose a medicine that is affordable, which in general benefits the patients, without harming them. Table 6 shows the sad consequences of the large NNH and NNH_{total} numbers of the chemical medicine in the long run, and Table 7 shows the danger of using drugs as medicine. As one of three patients are harmed every year with pharmaceutical drugs, and treatment often continues for life when the patient is not cured, the consequence is that almost every patient is harmed in the end, and 50 patients are harmed for every single, chronic patient helped or cured.

As one in 300 patients dies from the treatment with drugs every year, and effect seems to accumulate though time, a life-long treatment with drugs I likely to shorten your life with 10 years or more. It is estimated that in Denmark alone around 3000 patients are killed every year by the chemical medicine [23].

In Denmark over 2 million chronic patients out of a population of 5 millions uses drugs for about 6 billion Euros pr. Year (or 2-3,000 EURO per chronically ill patient, confirming the prize of drugs used in table 3). It is clear for us that the same money spent on the most efficient types of non-drug CAM [group 3, 4, 6, 8] would do immensely more for the population's health.

As this is not new, one wonders why chemical medicine is so much used, and why mind-body medicine is not part of the official health system.

Table 7. Accumulated harm and mortality caused by treatment (compared to non-treated, including live-saving effects of drugs) through time (year one, ten and fifty) for 10 classes of evidence-based medicine-prize for one patient cured

Continuous treatment (only stopped if the patient gets cured)	Number of patients cured for one patient harmed	Death including suicides (number of patients cured per patient killed by treatment)		
	Self-rated health	per cured patient	per cured patient	per cured patient
	NNH_{total}	First year	Year 10	Year 50
Medicine with drugs Class 1 – Chemical medicine	3	1-3	0.1-0.3	0.02-0.06
Class 2-CAM (Chemical CAM)	25	∞	∞	∞
Non-drug CAM				
Class 3a-CAM (Physical therapy, Low E)	1,000,000	∞	∞	∞
Class 3b-CAM (Physical therapy, High E.)	1,000	∞	∞	∞
Class 4-CAM (Psychotherapy)	1,000,000	∞	∞	∞
Class 5-CAM (Spiritual therapy)	1,000,000	∞	∞	∞
Class 6-CAM (Mind-Body medicine)	1,000,000	∞	∞	∞
Class 7–CAM Body-Spirit medicine	1,000,000	∞	∞	∞
Class 8-CAM (Holistic mind-body medicine)	1,000,000	∞	∞	∞
Class 9-CAM (Shamanism w. drugs)	1,000	∞	∞	∞
Class 10-CAM (Social/environm. medicine)	1,000,000	∞	∞	∞

One likely explanation is the close connection between pharmaceutical industry, the physicians and the public health system – often called the "medico-industrial complex".

This system is often seen to actively work against CAM, repressing CAM researchers and effectively by all means keeping CAM out of the political scene [20].

Drugs obviously turn patients into chronic patients instead of curing them. Half the population of the western world today is chronically ill, seemingly because of strong political and financial interests in biomedicine, leading to massive oppression of CAM in favor of drugs.

The shift from drugs to CAM would improve health radically in the society and reduce the cost of healthcare to a small fraction. Strict laws should be introduced immediately in all countries to stop the pharmaceutical industry and its collaborates from promoting drugs without evidence of therapeutic value (the ratio benefits: harm larger being no less than 1) and long term effect and patient safety, and from repressing CAM.

Conclusion

Strong economic and political interests seem to control medicine in Denmark and many other countries, making the pharmaceutical drugs often used, in spite of better and safer alternative for almost all clinical conditions (see [3, 10] for comprehensive lists of clinical conditions that can be helped or cured with mind-body medicine).

People who still doubt the reality of the low cost, high efficacy and safety of CAM presented in this review are encouraged to study Dean Ornish cure for coronary heart disease. It was this well-documented CAM cure for a serious disease that made us believe in the potentials of CAM [21, 22].

People who still doubt that pharmaceuticals often do more harm than good are encouraged to read the new book on the subject from the leader of the Nordic Cochrane Center Peter Gøtzsche [23], who concluded that "Our citizens would be far better of, if we removed all psychopharmacological drugs from the market, because the medical doctors are unable to handle them… Since they do more harm than good" [24].

We have seen that the 10 different types of evidence-based medicine have very different profiles when it comes to efficacy, cost pr. cured patient, cost per QALY, cost per HALY, and cost in harm on patients. In general chemical medicine, biomedicine as well as CAM, is expensive and harmful in the long run, while CAM i.e., massage therapy and psychotherapy is safe.

The best types of CAM, like mind-body medicine, holistic mind-body medicine (i.e., the classical Hippocratic medicine, often called clinical holistic medicine/CHM) are 50,000 times less harmful and 100 times more efficient in producing health and happiness (quality of life). The cost of one cured chronic patient is about 1,000,000€ with pharmaceutical drugs and 100,000€ or less with the efficient types of CAM.

Surprisingly we found pre-modern medicine – shamanism – to win the race in the end. While the drugs used often have some rare adverse effects, the efficacy of traditional one-session healing might make shamanistic medicine the cheapest, safest and most effective in the end. While we do not advocate the back-propagation to pre-modern times, we find it very interesting that such a medicine exists, inspiring us all to continue our quest for a still better medicine.

Acknowledgments

The Danish Quality of Life Survey, Quality of Life Research Center and the Research Clinic for Holistic Medicine, Copenhagen, was from 1987 till today supported by grants from the 1991 Pharmacy Foundation, the Goodwill-fonden, the JL-Foundation, E Danielsen and Wife's Foundation, Emmerick Meyer's Trust, the Frimodt-Heineken Foundation, the Hede Nielsen Family Foundation, Petrus Andersens Fond, Wholesaler CP Frederiksens Study Trust, Else and MogensWedell-Wedellsborg's Foundation and IMK Almene Fond. The research in quality of life and scientific complementary and holistic medicine was approved by the Copenhagen Scientific Ethical Committee under the numbers (KF)V. 100.1762-90, (KF)V. 100.2123/91, (KF)V. 01-502/ 93, (KF)V. 01-026/97, (KF)V. 01-162/97, (KF)V. 01-198/97, and further correspondence. We declare no conflicts of interest.

References

[1] Ventegodt, S., Merrick, S. Developing NCCAMs five category system for CAM into a new 10 class categorical system for all types of

medicine, based on four levels of human existence: molecules, body, mind and spirit. In preparation.

[2] Fontanarosa, P., Lundberg, G. Alternative medicine meets science. *JAMA* 1998; 280:1618-9.

[3] Ventegodt, S., Andersen, N. J., Kandel, I., Merrick, J. Comparative analysis of cost-effectiveness of non-drug medicine (non-pharmaceutical holistic, complementary and alternative medicine/CAM) and biomedicine (pharmaceutical drugs) for all clinical conditions. *Int. J. Disabil. Hum. Dev.* 2009;8(3):245-56.

[4] Ventegodt, S., Merrick, J. Therapeutic value (TV) of treatments with pharmaceutical drugs. Rough estimates for all clinical conditions based on Cochrane reviews and the ratio: Number Needed to Harm/Number Needed to Treat (TV=NNH_{total}/NNT). *BMJ* 2010 Nov. 15. URL: http://www.bmj.com/content/341/bmj.c5715.full/reply#bmj_el_244738.

[5] Ventegodt, S., Merrick, J. Therapeutic value (TV) of alternative medicine (non-drug CAM). Rough estimates for all clinical conditions based on Cochrane reviews and the ratio: Number Needed to Harm/ Number Needed to Treat (TV=NNH_{total}/NNT). *BMJ* 2010 Nov. 15. URL:http://www.bmj.com/content/341/bmj.c5715.full/reply#bmj_el_24 4740.

[6] Ventegodt, S., Merrick, J. A Review of side effects and adverse events of non-drug medicine (nonpharmaceutical complementary and alternative medicine): Psychotherapy, mind-body medicine and clinical holistic medicine. *J. Complement. Integr. Med.* 2009;6(1):16.

[7] National Center of Complementary and Alternative Medicine. URL: http://nccam.nih.gov/

[8] Committee on the Use of Complementary and Alternative Medicine by the American Public. Complementary and Alternative Medicine (CAM) in the United States. Washington, DC: National Academies Press, 2005.

[9] National Center for Complementary and Alternative Medicine. *Massage therapy: AnIntroduction.* Bethesda, MD:NCCAM Publication No. D327, 2006.

[10] Ventegodt, S., Omar, H., Merrick, J. Quality of life as medicine: Interventions that induce salutogenesis. A review of the literature. *Soc. Indicat. Res.* 2009. DOI: 10.1007/s11205-010-9621-8.

[11] Ventegodt, S., Thegler, S., Andreasen, T., Struve, F., Enevoldsen, L., Bassaine, L., et al. Clinical holistic medicine: Psychodynamic short-time therapy complemented with bodywork. A clinical follow-up study of 109 patients. *Scientific World Journal* 2006;6:2220-38.

[12] Ventegodt, S., Hermansen, T. D., Flensborg-Madsen, T., Nielsen, M. L., Clausen, B., Merrick, J. Human development V: biochemistry unable to explain the emergence of biological form (morphogenesis) and therefore a new principle as source of biological information is needed. *Scientific World Journal* 2006; 6:1359-67.

[13] Lazarou, J., Pomeranz, B. H., Corey, P. N. Incidence of adverse drug reactions in hospitalized patients: a meta-analysis of prospective studies. *JAMA* 1998; 279(15):1200-5.

[14] Ventegodt, S. *Quality of life in Denmark. Results from a population survey*. Copenhagen: Forskningscentrets Forlag, 1995.

[15] Long, M. J., McQueen, D. A., Banga-lore, V. G., Schurman, J. R. 2nd. Using self-assessed health to predict patient outcomes after total knee replacement. *Clin. Orthop. Relat. Res.* 2005; 434:189-92.

[16] Idler, E. L., Russell, L. B., Davis, D. Survival, functional limitations, and self-rated health in the NHANES I epidemiologic follow-up study, 1992. First national health and nutrition examination survey. *Am. J. Epidemiol.* 2000; 152 (9):874-83.

[17] Idler, E. L., Kasl, S. Health perceptions and survival: do global evaluations of health status really predict mortality? *J. Gerontol.* 1991; 46(2):S55-65.

[18] Burström, B., Fredlund, P. Self rated health: Is it as good a predictor of subsequent mortality among adults in lower as well as in higher social classes. *J. Epidemiol. Community Health* 2001;55(11):836-40.

[19] Grof, S. *LSD psychotherapy: Exploring the frontiers of the hidden mind*. Alameda, CA: Hunter House, 1980.

[20] Ventegodt, S., Andersen, N. J., Kandel, I. Bio- and alternative medicine in conflict. Human rights protection of the alternative therapist. *J. Altern. Med. Res.* 2009;1(2):189-202.

[21] Ornish, D., Brown, S. E., Scherwitz, L. W., Billings, J. H., Armstrong, W. T., et al. Can lifestyle changes reverse coronary heart disease? The lifestyle heart trial. *Lancet* 1990; 336(8708):129-33.

[22] Ornish, D., Scherwitz, L. W., Billings, J. H., Brown, S. E., Gould, K. L., et al. Intensive lifestyle changes for reversal of coronary heart disease. *JAMA* 1998; 280(23):2001-7.

[23] Gøtzsche, P. C., Smith, R., Rennie, D. *Deadly medicines and organised crime: How big pharma has corrupted healthcare*. London: Radcliffe, 2013.

[24] Gøtzsche, P. C. [Psykiatri på afveje. Vi ville være langt bedre stillet, hvis alle psykofarmaka blev fjernet fra markedet. Lægerne er ikke i stand til at håndtere dem]. *Politiken* 2014 Jan. 06 [Danish].

Bibliography

50 studies every doctor should know: the key studies that form the foundation of evidence based medicine LCCN: 2013017001 Type of material: Book Main title: 50 studies every doctor should know: the key studies that form the foundation of evidence based medicine/edited by Michael E. Hochman, M.D., MPH. Edition: Revised edition. Published/Created: Oxford; New York: Oxford University Press, [2014] Description: xvii, 323 pages: illustrations; 24 cm ISBN: 9780199343560 (pbk.: alk. paper) 9780199343577 (alk. paper) 9780199343584 (alk. paper) LC classification: R853.C55 A155 2014 Variant title: Fifty studies every doctor should know Related names: Hochman, Michael E. Subjects: Biomedical Research--Abstracts. Evaluation Studies as Topic--Abstracts. Evidence-Based Medicine--Abstracts. Notes: Includes bibliographical references and index. Dewey class no.: 610.72/4 NLM class no.: ZW 20.5 Other system no.: (DNLM)101606852 Shelf Location: FLM2014 109404 CALL NUMBER: R853.C55 A155 2014 OVERFLOWA5S Request in: Jefferson or Adams Building Reading Rooms (FLM1)

50 studies every internist should know LCCN: 2014043394 Type of material: Book Main title: 50 studies every internist should know/edited by Kristopher Swiger, Joshua R. Thomas, Michael E. Hochman, Steven Hochman. Published/Produced: Oxford; New York: Oxford University Press, [2014] Projected pub date: 1501 Description: p.; cm. ISBN: 9780199349937 (alk. paper) LC

classification: RC46 Variant title: Fifty studies every internist should know Related names: Swiger, Kristopher, editor. Thomas, Joshua R., editor. Hochman, Michael E., editor. Hochman, Steven, editor. Subjects: Internal Medicine--methods. Evidence-Based Medicine. Preventive Medicine--methods. Notes: Includes bibliographical references and index. Series: 50 studies every doctor should know 50 studies every doctor should know (Series) Dewey class no.: 616 NLM class no.: WB 115 Other system no.: (DNLM)101645171 Content type: text Media type: unmediated Carrier type: volume

A systematic process to facilitate evidence-informed decisionmaking regarding program expansion LCCN: 2013371137 Type of material: Book Personal name: Martin, Laurie T. (Laurie Thayer), 1974- author. Main title: A systematic process to facilitate evidence-informed decisionmaking regarding program expansion/Laurie T. Martin, Coreen Farris, David M. Adamson, Robin M. Weinick. Published/Produced: Santa Monica, CA: Rand Corporation, [2014] ©2014 Description: xvi, 70 pages: illustrations; 28 cm. Links: Electronic Version: Publisher's web page for this work, including abstract, table of contents, and link to scanned depiction of full text: http://www.rand.org/pubs/research_reports/RR487z3.html ISBN: 9780833084170 (pbk.) 0833084178 (pbk.) Related names: Farris, Coreen, author. Adamson, David M., author. Weinick, Robin M., author. Rand Corporation, issuing body. National Defense Research Institute (U.S.), issuing body. Subjects: Medical care--United States--Evaluation. Mental health services--United States--Evaluation. Brain--Wounds and injuries--Treatment--Evaluation. Health services administration--United States. Evidence-based medicine--Handbooks, manuals, etc. Notes: "RAND Corporation research report series."--Web page (PDF). "Prepared for the Office of the Secretary of Defense and the Defense Centers of Excellence for Psychological Health and Traumatic Brain Injury."--Title page. "National Defense Research Institute." "RR-487/3-OSD."--Page 4 of printed paper wrapper. "Approved for public release; distribution unlimited."--Title page. "Glossary": pages xv-xvi. Includes bibliographical references (pages 69-70). "This research was sponsored ... under Contract W74V8H-06-C-0002."--Verso of title page. Series: RAND toolkit; v. 3 RAND toolkit; v. 3. Report no. RR-487/3-OSD Geographic area code: n-us--- Other system no.: (OCoLC)ocn867840220 Content type: text Media type: unmediated Carrier type: volume CALL NUMBER: Not available Request in: Jefferson or Adams Building Reading Rooms

Acupuncture and moxibustion as an evidence-based therapy for cancer LCCN: 2012947032 Type of material: Book Main title: Acupuncture and moxibustion as an evidence-based therapy for cancer/William C.S. Cho, editor. Published/Produced: Dordrecht: Springer, c2012. Description: xi, 354 p.: ill.; 24 cm. ISBN: 9789400748323 (alk. paper) 9400748329 (alk. paper) 9789400748330 (ebook) 9400748337 (ebook) LC classification: RC271.A62 A28 2012 Related names: Cho, William C. S. Subjects: Cancer--Alternative treatment. Acupuncture. Moxa. Evidence-based medicine. Neoplasms--therapy. Acupuncture Therapy. Evidence-Based Medicine. Moxibustion. Notes: Includes bibliographical references and index. Series: Evidence-based anticancer complementary and alternative medicine, 2211-0534; v. 3 Evidence-based anticancer complementary and alternative medicine; 3. 2211-0534 Dewey class no.: 616.99/406 NLM class no.: 2013 A-697 QZ 266 National bib agency no.: 101600862 016240145 Other system no.: (OCoLC)ocn796763042 Shelf Location: FLM2014 124932 CALL NUMBER: RC271.A62 A28 2012 OVERFLOWA5S Request in: Jefferson or Adams Building Reading Rooms (FLM1)

AMA Guides to the evaluation of disease and injury causation LCCN: 2013017371 Type of material: Book Uniform title: Guides to the evaluation of disease and injury causation Main title: AMA Guides to the evaluation of disease and injury causation/[edited by] J. Mark Melhorn, James B. Talmage, William E. Ackerman III, Mark H. Hyman. Edition: Second edition. Published/Produced: Chicago, Illinois: American Medical Association, [2014] Description: xxiv, 792 pages; 26 cm ISBN: 9781603598682 (pbk.: alk. paper) LC classification: RC963.4 .G82 2014 Related names: Melhorn, J.

Mark, editor of compilation. Talmage, James B., editor of compilation. Ackerman, William E., III, editor of compilation. Hyman, Mark H., editor of compilation. American Medical Association, issuing body. Summary: "The second edition of AMA Guides to the Evaluation of Disease and Injury Causation is dedicated to updating the science, expanding the focus, and including additional perspectives to improve the understanding of causation, which will eventually improve the treatment outcomes for the injured worker as they stay-at-home or return-to-work"--Provided by publisher. Subjects: Occupational Diseases--etiology. Disability Evaluation. Evidence-Based Medicine--methods. Occupational Diseases--diagnosis. Occupational Exposure. Occupational Injuries--etiology. Notes: Includes bibliographical references and index. Dewey class no.: 616.07/5 NLM class no.: WA 400 Other system no.: (DNLM)101607012 Content type: text Media type: unmediated Carrier type: volume Shelf Location: FLM2014 069825 CALL NUMBER: RC963.4 .G82 2014 OVERFLOWA5S Request in: Jefferson or Adams Building Reading Rooms (FLM1) CALL NUMBER: RC963.4 .G82 2014 Copy 2 Request in: Reference - Science Reading Room (Adams, 5th Floor)

An introduction to evidence-based practice in nursing & healthcare LCCN: 2011022071 Type of material: Book Personal name: Pooler, Alison. Main title: An introduction to evidence-based practice in nursing & healthcare/Alison Pooler. Published/Created: Harlow, England: Pearson, c2012. Description: iv, 92 p.: ill.; 22 cm. ISBN: 9780273722953 (pbk.) LC classification: R723.7 .P66 2012 Variant title: An introduction to evidence-based practice in nursing and healthcare Contents: What is research? -- What is evidence and evidence-based practice? -- Why do we need evidence base in our clinical practice? -- Clinical guidelines and the need for clinical audit -- Change management in the implementation of evidence-based practice. Subjects: Evidence-based medicine. Evidence-Based Practice. Notes: Includes bibliographical references (p. 82-83) and index. Dewey class no.: 610.73 NLM class no.: WB 102.5 Other system no.: (DNLM)101561226 CALL NUMBER: R723.7 .P66 2012 Copy 1 Request in: Jefferson or Adams Building Reading Rooms

Applied topics in health psychology LCCN: 2012017996 Type of material: Book Main title: Applied topics in health psychology/edited by Marie L. Caltabiano and Lina A. Ricciardelli. Published/Created: Chichester, West Sussex, UK; Malden, MA, USA: Wiley-Blackwell, 2013. Description: xxx, 528 p.: ill.; 25 cm. ISBN: 9781119971931 (pbk.) LC classification: RA776.9 .A67 2013 Related names: Caltabiano, Marie L., 1959- Ricciardelli, Lina A. Subjects: Health behavior. Well-being. Health attitudes--Australia. Health promotion--Australia. Health Behavior--Australia. Attitude to Health--Australia. Behavioral Medicine--Australia. Evidence-Based Medicine--Australia. Notes: Includes bibliographical references and index. Dewey class no.: 616.8900994 Geographic area code: u-at--- NLM class no.: W 85 Other system no.: (DNLM)101583488 Shelf Location: FLM2014 026185 CALL NUMBER: RA776.9 .A67 2013 OVERFLOWA5S Request in: Jefferson or Adams Building Reading Rooms (FLM1)

Auditory processing disorders: assessment, management, and treatment LCCN: 2012032011 Type of material: Book Main title: Auditory processing disorders: assessment, management, and treatment/[edited by] Donna Geffner and Deborah Ross-Swain. Edition: 2nd ed. Published/Created: San Diego: Plural Pub., c2013. Description: xix, 883 p.: ill.; 26 cm. ISBN: 9781597564953 (alk. paper) 1597564958 (alk. paper) LC classification: RC394.W63 A94 2013 Related names: Geffner, Donna S. Ross-Swain, Deborah. Subjects: Auditory Perceptual Disorders--therapy. Auditory Perceptual Disorders--diagnosis. Evidence-Based Medicine. Notes: Includes bibliographical references and index. Dewey class no.: 617.8 NLM class no.: WV 270 Other system no.: (DNLM)101590110 CALL NUMBER: RC394.W63 A94 2013 Copy 2 Request in: Jefferson or Adams Building Reading Rooms Shelf Location: FLM2014 020529 CALL NUMBER: RC394.W63 A94 2013 OVERFLOWA5S Request in: Jefferson or Adams Building Reading Rooms (FLM1)

Autism spectrum disorder: a clinical guide for general practitioners LCCN: 2013017833 Type of material: Book Personal name: Durand, Vincent Mark. Main title: Autism spectrum disorder: a clinical guide for general practitioners/V. Mark Durand. Edition: First Edition. Published/Produced: Washington, DC: American Psychological Association, [2014] Description: x, 183 pages; 24 cm ISBN: 9781433815690 1433815699 LC classification: RC553.A88 D86 2014 Contents: Autism spectrum disorder: background and cases -- Diagnostic criteria and epidemiology -- Etiology -- Comorbid conditions -- Screening, diagnosis, and assessment -- Treatment -- Addressing the needs of family members. Subjects: Autism spectrum disorders. Autism spectrum disorders in children. Evidence-based medicine. Notes: Includes bibliographical references (pages 133-169) and index. Dewey class no.: 616.85/882 Content type: text Media type: unmediated Carrier type: volume Shelf Location: FLM2014 015987 CALL NUMBER: RC553.A88 D86 2014 OVERFLOWA5S Request in: Jefferson or Adams Building Reading Rooms (FLM1) CALL NUMBER: RC553.A88 D86 2014 Copy 2 Request in: Reference - Science Reading Room (Adams, 5th Floor)

Becoming a consummate clinician: what every student, house officer, and hospital practitioner needs to know LCCN: 2012023634 Type of material: Book Personal name: Goldberger, Ary Louis, 1949- Main title: Becoming a consummate clinician: what every student, house officer, and hospital practitioner needs to know/Ary L. Goldberger, Zachary D. Goldberger. Published/Created: Hoboken, N.J.: Wiley-Blackwell, c2012. Description: xii, 210 p.: ill.; 24 cm. ISBN: 9781118011430 (pbk.) LC classification: R690 .G65 2012 Related names: Goldberger, Zachary D. Summary: "The Consummate Clinician offers hospital-based physicians an organizing framework for coping with daily challenges both in patient care and in teaching. The book describes in a highly formatted, easily accessible way exactly how physicians and physicians-in-training can think critically and act decisively in this age of medical information overload. Special emphasis is on (1) error avoidance and reduction - a topic that has long been championed by hospitalists, (2) efficient practice management for best patient outcomes and improved cost control, (3) the use of evidence-based medicine, and (4) improving communication among and between physicians and other staff in the hospital setting. Using real-world clinical examples and scenarios, the book focuses on essential topics, many of which tend to fall between the cracks of print and electronic resources. Pearls and pitfalls of gathering, processing, and communicating medical information are presented, but more than these, this book is meant as a kind of clinical GPS--a way of helping hospital-based physicians find their clinical coordinates and keep their bearings in the face of new challenges and uncertainties. In addition to the clinical scenarios featured throughout, additional mini-cases are collected at the end of the book. The over-arching goal of this new resource is to enrich the way hospital-based physicians think about diagnosis, therapy, and prognosis, especially at the warp-speed of "ward world," which increasingly lurches between the frazzled and the frantic"--Provided by publisher. Subjects: Clinical Medicine. Evidence-Based Medicine. Interprofessional Relations. Medical Errors--prevention & control. Teaching Rounds--methods. Notes: Includes bibliographical references and index. Series: Hospital medicine: current concepts; 3 Dewey class no.: 610.73 NLM class no.: WB 102 Other system no.: (DNLM)101586060 Shelf Location: FLM2013 003298 CALL NUMBER: R690 .G65 2012 OVERFLOWA5S Request in: Jefferson or Adams Building Reading Rooms (FLM1) CALL NUMBER: R690 .G65 2012 LANDOVR Copy 2 Request in: Jefferson or Adams Building Reading Rooms - STORED OFFSITE

Best evidence for spine surgery
LCCN: 2011045627 Type of material: Book Main title: Best evidence for spine surgery/editors, Rahul Jandial, Steven R. Garfin; associate editors, Christopher Ames ... [et al.]. Edition: 1st ed. Published/Created: Philadelphia: Elsevier/Saunders, c2012. Projected pub date: 1202 Description: p.; cm. ISBN: 9781437716252 (hardcover: alk. paper) Related names: Jandial, Rahul. Garfin, Steven R. Ames, Christopher P. Contents:

Cervical disk herniation: anterior cervical diskectomy and fusion versus arthroplasty/Mir H. Ali, Frank M. Phillips -- Multilevel anterior cervical diskectomy and fusion: bone-grafting options/Sheeraz A. Qureshi, Andrew C. Hecht, Scott D. Boden -- Ossification of the posterior longitudinal ligament: anterior versus posterior approach/Garrick W. Cason, Edward R. Anderson III, Harry N. Herkowitz -- Minimally invasive approaches to thoracic disk herniations/Alfred T. Ogden, Michael G. Kaiser, Richard G. Fessler -- Lumbar disk herniation with mild neurological deficit: microdiskectomy versus conservative treatment/Kelli L. Crabtree, Paul M. Arnold -- Cervical spondylosis-spinal stenosis: laminoplasty versus laminectomy and fusion/Yu-Po Lee, Niraj Patel, Steven R. Garfin -- Lumbar degenerative disk disease: fusion versus artificial disk/Michael F. Duffy, Jack E. Zigler -- Degenerative spondylolisthesis with radicular pain: decompression only versus decompression and fusion/Tuan V. Nguyen, Robert A. McGuire Jr. -- Asymptomatic intradural Schwannoma: surgery versus radiosurgery versus observation/Christopher E. Mandigo, Paul C. McCormick -- Pseudotumor: transoral versus posterior fusion/Daniel M. Sciubba ... [et al.] -- Odontoid fracture in the elderly: odontoid screws versus posterior fusion/Harvey E. Smith, Scott D. Daffner, Alexander R. Vaccaro -- C1-C2 fusion: transarticular screws versus Harms procedure/Thomas J. Kesman, Bradford L. Currier -- Multilevel cervical corpectomy: anterior-only versus circumferential instrumentation/Andrew J. Schoenfeld, Christopher M. Bono -- Cervical jumped facets and incomplete neurological deficit: closed reduction versus urgent surgery/Michael A. Finn, Paul A. Anderson -- Laminectomy across cervico thoracic junction: fusion versus non fusion/Timothy E. Link, Rahul Jandial, Volker K.H. Sonntag -- Vertebral metastases: ventral and dorsal approach versus lateral -- Extracavitary transpedicular approach/John H. Shin, Edward C. Benzel -- Degenerative scoliosis: anterior and posterior fusion versus posterior fusion/Krishna Gumidyala, Sigurd Berven -- Sagittal imbalance: multiple Smith-Petersen osteotomies versus pedicle substraction osteotomies/Jamal McClendon ... [et al.] -- -- L1-S1 fusion:

extending to T12 and pelvis and when to include L5-S1 anterior grafting/Steven Mardjetko -- High-grade spondylolisthesis: reduction and fusion versus in situ fusion/Matthew B. Maserati, Christopher I. Shaffrey, Adam S. Kanter. Subjects: Spine--surgery--Case Reports. Evidence-Based Medicine--Case Reports. Orthopedic Procedures--methods--Case Reports. Spinal Diseases--surgery--Case Reports. Notes: Includes bibliographical references and index. Dewey class no.: 617.5/6059 NLM class no.: WE 725 Other system no.: (DNLM)101572366

Best evidence structural interventions for HIV prevention LCCN: 2013937048 Type of material: Book Personal name: Golden, Rachel E., author. Main title: Best evidence structural interventions for HIV prevention/Rachel E. Golden, Charles B. Collins, Shayna D. Cunningham, Emily N. Newman, Josefina J. Card. Published/Produced: New York, NY: Springer, [2013] ©2013 Description: viii, 352 pages; 25 cm ISBN: 9781461470120 (hbk) 1461470129 (hbk) LC classification: RA643.8 .G64 2013 Related names: Collins, Charles B., author. Cunningham, Shayna, author. Newman, Emily N., author. Card, Josefina J., author. Contents: Overview of structural interventions to decrease injection drug-use risk -- Overview of structural interventions to decrease noncommercial sex risk -- Overview of structural interventions to decrease commercial sex risk -- Overview of structural interventions to increase voluntary counseling and testing (VCT) and antiretroviral therapy (ART). Subjects: HIV infections--Prevention. AIDS (Disease)--Prevention. HIV Infections--prevention & control. Evidence-Based Medicine. AIDS (Disease)--Prevention. HIV infections--Prevention. Notes: Includes bibliographical references and index. NLM class no.: 2013 H-571 WC 503.6 National bib agency no.: 016294912 101615846 Other system no.: (OCoLC)ocn828892007 Invalid ISBN: 9781461470137 (eBook) Content type: text Media type: unmediated Carrier type: volume CALL NUMBER: RA643.8 .G64 2013 Copy 1 Request in: Jefferson or Adams Building Reading Rooms

Brain, mind, and developmental psychopathology in childhood

LCCN: 2011046406 Type of material: Book Main title: Brain, mind, and developmental psychopathology in childhood/edited by Elena Garralda and Jean-Philippe Raynaud. Published/Created: Lanham, Md: Jason Aronson, 2012. Projected pub date: 1111 Description: p.; cm. ISBN: 9780765708649 (cloth: alk. paper) 9780765708656 (paper: alk. paper) 9780765708663 (electronic) Related names: Garralda, M. Elena. Raynaud, Jean-Philippe, 1960- Summary: "Brain, Mind, and Developmental Psychopathology in Childhood, part of the International Association of Child and Adolescent Psychiatry and Allied Professions' book series "Working with Children & Adolescents" edited by Elena Garralda and Jean-Philippe Raynaud updates the knowledge about connections between brain, mind, and developmental psychopathology. The volume illuminates our understanding of different types of psychiatric disorders in children including autism, hyperkinetic disorder, obsessive compulsive disorder, and childhood schizophreniaand the effects of child maltreatment and deliberate self harm. This book describes how to integrate physical and psychological treatments for child and adolescent mental health problems and advocacy for the treatment of children and adolescents with mental health problems. "--Provided by publisher. Contents: Machine generated contents note: IACAPAP Book Series -- Acknowledgments -- About the Contributors -- Preface, by Olayinka Omigbodun -- Editorial Introduction, by M Elena Garralda & Jean-Philippe Raynaud -- Part I: Biological and Psychological Influences on Developmental Psychopathology -- The Developmental Being: Modeling a Probabilistic Approach to Child Development and Psychopathology, by David Cohen -- Antecedents in Infancy of Personality Disorders: The Interplay Between Biological and Psychological Processes, by Miri Keren and Sam Tyano -- Insights into Childhood Psychiatric Disorders from Developmental Neuro-imaging, by Philip Shaw -- Common and Rare Genetic Variants as Risk Factors for Autism Spectrum Disorders, by Marie Christine Mouren, Thomas Bourgeron, Richard Delorme -- Part II: Individual Disorders/Problems: Updates -- Obsessive-Compulsive Disorder, by Luisa Lazaro and Josep Toro -- The

Relationship Between Autism and Schizophrenia: A Reappraisal, by Saskia Palmen and Herman van Engeland -- Early-onset Schizophrenia, by Helmut Remschmidt and Frank Theisen -- Developmental Dyslexia, by Andreas Warnke, Gerd Schulte-Korne & Elena Ise -- Chapter 9: Effects of Child Maltreatment on the Developing Brain, by Dayna Glaser -- Self-Harm in Adolescents, by Dennis Ougrin, Troy Tranah, Eleanor Leigh, Lucy Taylor and Joan R. Asarnow -- Part IV: Treatment and Advocacy -- Integrating Medical and Psychological Therapies in Child Mental Health: An Evidence Based Medicine Approach, by Jeffrey J. Sapyta and John S. March -- Learning Disorders, by Daniel Fung & Liying Su -- Advocacy for Child and Adolescent Mental Health, by Gordon Harper. Subjects: Mental Disorders--psychology. Adolescent. Child Development. Child. Mental Disorders--etiology. Psychopathology. Notes: Includes bibliographical references and index. Series: IACAPAP book series IACAPAP book series. The working with children and adolescents series IACAPAP book series; v. 19. IACAPAP book series. The working with children and adolescents series. Dewey class no.: 618.92/89 NLM class no.: WS 350.6 Other system no.: (DNLM)101572599 CALL NUMBER: Not available Request in: Jefferson or Adams Building Reading Rooms

Breastfeeding management for the clinician: using the evidence LCCN: 2013012434 Type of material: Book Personal name: Walker, Marsha. Main title: Breastfeeding management for the clinician: using the evidence/Marsha Walker. Edition: 3rd ed. Published/Created: Burlington, MA: Jones & Bartlett Learning, c2014. Description: ix, 626 p.: ill.; 23 cm. ISBN: 9781449694654 (pbk.) LC classification: RJ216 .W339 2014 Contents: Influence of the biospecificity of human milk -- Influence of the maternal anatomy and physiology on lactation -- Influence of the infant's anatomy and physiology -- Influence of peripartum factors, birthing practices, and early caretaking behaviors -- First 24-48 hours: common challenges -- Beyond the initial 48-72 hours: infant challenges -- Physical, medical, and environmental problems and issues -- Maternal pathology: breast and nipple issues --

Physical, medical, emotional, and environmental challenges to the breastfeeding mother. Subjects: Breast Feeding. Evidence-Based Medicine. Lactation--physiology. Notes: Includes bibliographical references and index. Dewey class no.: 649/.33 NLM class no.: WS 125 Other system no.: (DNLM)101604920 Shelf Location: FLM2013 028754 CALL NUMBER: RJ216 .W339 2014 OVERFLOWA5S Request in: Jefferson or Adams Building Reading Rooms (FLM1)

Cardiopulmonary physical therapy: management and case studies LCCN: 2013023319 Type of material: Book Personal name: Reid, W. Darlene, author. Uniform title: Clinical management notes and case histories in cardiopulmonary physical therapy Main title: Cardiopulmonary physical therapy: management and case studies/W. Darlene Reid, Frank Chung, Kylie Hill. Edition: Second edition. Published/Produced: Thorofare, NJ: Slack Incorporated, [2014] Description: xxii, 469 pages; 26 cm. ISBN: 9781617110290 (hardback: alk. paper) LC classification: RC702 .R455 2014 Related names: Chung, Frank, author. Hill, Kylie, 1973- author. Summary: "Cardiopulmonary Physical Therapy: Management and Case Studies, Second Edition is a unique and succinct textbook for the classroom that blends clinical notes on assessment and management together with case-based instructional approaches to cardiopulmonary care for acute and ambulatory care patients. This one-of-a-kind text describes current approaches that cover traditional physical therapist management strategies and includes evidence-based chapters on early mobilization and exercise training on a wide range of cardiopulmonary patient groups. The updated Second Edition presents twenty-four cases that were designed to complement each chapter topic and represent the most common pulmonary, cardiac, and neurological conditions that are typically managed in cardiopulmonary care. These cases have been carefully selected and developed over several years to illustrate a spectrum of clinical issues essential for the preparation of the entry-level therapist. The very interactive nature of the case history approach is engaging and provides the opportunity to work through many of the steps of the clinical decision-making process. Cardiopulmonary Physical Therapy: Management and Case Studies, Second Edition also includes answer guides for the questions posed in the assessment and management chapters, as well as for the twenty-four cases. The two-fold evidence and case-based learning approach used by Dr. W. Darlene Reid, Frank Chung, and Dr. Kylie Hill allows for a more engaging experience. The inclusion of interactive materials will allow students to learn and develop skills to prepare themselves for their professional transition while clinicians can use the text as a reference tool"--Provided by publisher. Subjects: Respiratory Tract Diseases--rehabilitation--Case Reports. Evidence-Based Medicine--Case Reports. Heart Diseases--rehabilitation--Case Reports. Physical Therapy Modalities--Case Reports. Notes: Preceded by Clinical management notes and case histories in cardiopulmonary physical therapy/W. Darlene Reid, Frank Chung. 2004. Includes bibliographical references and index. Dewey class no.: 616.2/0046 NLM class no.: WF 145 Other system no.: (DNLM)101610153 Content type: text Media type: unmediated Carrier type: volume Shelf Location: FLM2014 019770 CALL NUMBER: RC702 .R455 2014 OVERFLOWA5S Request in: Jefferson or Adams Building Reading Rooms (FLM1)

Cardiovascular diseases: from molecular pharmacology to evidence-based therapeutics LCCN: 2014050157 Type of material: Book Personal name: Li, Yunbo, author. Main title: Cardiovascular diseases: from molecular pharmacology to evidence-based therapeutics/Y. Robert Li. Published/Produced: Hoboken, New Jersey: John Wiley & Sons, Inc., [2015] Projected pub date: 1505 Description: p.; cm. ISBN: 9780470915370 (cloth) LC classification: RM345 Subjects: Cardiovascular Diseases--drug therapy. Case Reports. Evidence-Based Medicine--methods. Molecular Medicine--methods. Notes: Includes index. Additional formats: Online version: Li, Yunbo, author. Cardiovascular diseases Hoboken, New Jersey: John Wiley & Sons, Inc., [2015] 9781118889916 (DLC) 2015000334 Dewey class no.: 616.1/061 NLM class no.: WG 166 Other system no.: (DNLM)101648918 Content type: text Media type: unmediated Carrier type: volume

Casebook of evidence-based therapy for eating disorders LCCN: 2014042003 Type of material: Book Main title: Casebook of evidence-based therapy for eating disorders/edited by Heather Thompson-Brenner. Published/Produced: New York: The Guilford Press, 2015. Projected pub date: 1506 Description: p.; cm. ISBN: 9781462520688 (hardcover: alk. paper) LC classification: RC552.E18 Related names: Thompson-Brenner, Heather, editor. Contents: Overcoming fear of eating: exposure and response prevention for anorexia nervosa/Deborah R. Glasofer, Anne Marie Albano, H. Blair Simpson, & Joanna E. Steinglass -- Family-based treatment for anorexia nervosa in adolescents/Angela Celio Doyle & Daniel Le Grange -- Enhancing motivation via text messaging: an adaptation of motivational interviewing for eating disorders/Rebecca M. Shingleton, Tibor P. Palfai, & Heather Thompson-Brenner -- Cognitive remediation therapy and cognitive-behavioral therapy with an older adult with anorexia nervosa/Alison M. Darcy, Kathleen K. Fitzpatrick, & James Lock -- Psychoanalytic psychotherapy for bulimia nervosa/Susanne Lunn, Stig Poulsen, & Sarah I. F. Daniel -- Emotion acceptance behavior therapy for anorexia nervosa/Jennifer E. Wildes, Marsha D. Marcus, & Elizabeth B. McCabe -- Interpersonal psychotherapy for the prevention of weight gain and eating disorders/Marian Tanofsky-Kraff, Lauren B. Shomaker, Jami F. Young, & Denise E. Wilfley -- Integrating couple-based interventions into the treatment of adult anorexia nervosa: a case example of ""UCAN""/Melanie S. Fischer, Jennifer S. Kirby, T. J. Raney, Cynthia M. Bulik, & Donald H. Baucom -- Cognitive behavior therapy for night eating syndrome/Jennifer D. Lundgren, Kelly C. Allison -- Enhanced cognitive-behavioral therapy-broad for complex bulimia nervosa/Heather Thompson-Brenner, Rebecca Shingleton, Dana Satir, & Elizabeth Pratt -- Dialectical behavior therapy for bulimia nervosa and major depressive disorder/Kay Segal, Lindsey A. Ohler, Kalina Eneva, & Eunice Chen -- Adolescent-focused therapy for anorexia nervosa/Kathleen Kara Fitzpatrick, Renee Rienecke Hoste, James Lock, & Daniel Le

Grange. Subjects: Eating Disorders--therapy. Cognitive Therapy--methods. Evidence-Based Medicine. Family Therapy--methods. Notes: Includes bibliographical references and index. Dewey class no.: 616.85/260651 NLM class no.: WM 175 Other system no.: (DNLM)101644234 Content type: text Media type: unmediated Carrier type: volume

Clinical decision support: the road to broad adoption LCCN: 2014434392 Type of material: Book Main title: Clinical decision support: the road to broad adoption/edited by Robert A. Greenes Edition: 2nd ed. Published/Created: Amsterdam: Boston: Academic Press, c2014. Description: xxxix, 887 p.: ill.; 24 cm. ISBN: 9780123984760 0123984769 Related names: Greenes, Robert A., 1940- edt Contents: Sect. 1: Computer-based clinical decision support: overview, status, and challenges. Ch. 1. Definition, scope and challenges/Robert A. Greenes -- Ch. 2. A brief history of clinical decision support/Robert A. Greenes -- Ch. 3. Features of computer-based clinical decision support/Robert A. Greenes -- Ch. 4. The role of quality measurement and reporting feedback as a driver for care improvement/Floyd Eisenberg -- Sect. 2: Experience with CDS development and adoption: case studies, national initiatives, and lessons learned. Ch. 5. Regenstrief medical informatics/Paul Biondich, [et al.] -- Ch. 6. Patients, doctors, and information technology: clinical decision support at Brigham and Women's Hospital and Partners HealthCare/Adam Wright and David W. Bates -- Ch. 7. Computer-based approaches to improving healthcare quality and safety at LDS Hospital/R. Scott Evans -- Ch. 8. International dimensions of clinical decision support/Hamish Fraser and Jeremy Wyatt -- Ch. 9. Current state of CDS utilization/Robert A. Greenes -- Sect. 3: Sources of knowledge for clinical decision support. Ch. 10. Human-intensive techniques/Vimla L. Patel and Edward H. Shortliffe -- Ch. 11. Generation of knowledge for clinical decision support/Michael E. Matheny and Lucila Ohno-Machado -- Ch. 12. Modernizing evidence synthesis for evidence-based medicine/Byron C. Wallace, [et al.] -- Ch. 13. Big data and population-based decision support/Michael A. Krall, Adi V. Gundlapalli and Matthew H. Samore -- Ch. 14. Clinical decision support for personalized medicine/Brandon M. Welch, [et al.]. Sect. 4: The technology of clinical decision support. Ch. 15. Decision rules and expressions/Robert A. Jenders -- Ch. 16. Guidelines and workflow models/Mor Peleg and Arturo González-Ferrer -- Ch. 17. Ontologies, vocabularies and data models/Stanley M. Huff, [et al.] -- Ch. 18. Grouped knowledge elements/Margarita Sordo and Aziz A. Boxwala -- Ch. 19. Infobuttons and point of care access to knowledge/Guilherme Del Fiol, Hong Yu and James J. Cimino -- Ch. 20. Formal representations and semantice web technologies/Alan Rector and Davide Sottara -- Ch. 21. The role of standards/Kensaku Kawamoto and Robert A. Greenes -- Sect. 5: Adoption of clinical decision support. Ch. 22. Cognitive considerations for health information technology/Amy Franklin and Jiajie Zhang -- Ch. 23. Organizational and cultural change/Joan S. Ash and Timothy H. Hartzog -- Ch. 24. Managing the investment in clinical decision support/John Glaser and Tonya Hongsermeier -- Ch. 25. A clinical decision support implementation guide: practical considerations/Donald Levick and Jerome Osheroff -- Ch. 26. Legal and regulatory issues related to the use of clinical software in health care delivery/Steven H. Brown and Randolph A. Miller -- Ch. 27. Consumers and clinical decision support/Nananda Col and Rosaly Correa-de-Araujo -- Sect. 6: The journey to widespread use of clinical decision support. Ch. 28. A clinical knowledge management program/Roberto A. Rocha, [et al.] -- Ch. 29. Integration of knowledge resources into applications to enable CDS/Kensaku Kawamoto, Emory Fry and Robert Greenes -- Ch. 30. Looking ahead: the road to broad adoption/Robert A. Greenes. Subjects: Diagnosis--Decision making--Data processing. Clinical medicine--Decision making--Data processing. Decision Support Systems, Clinical--trends Clinical Medicine--trends Delivery of Health Care--trends Medical Informatics Applications Problem Solving Clinical medicine--Decision making--Data processing. Diagnosis--Decision making--Data processing. Notes: Includes bibliographical references and index. Additional formats: Electronic book (OCoLC)875640465 National bib agency no.: 016747088 Other system no.: (OCoLC)ocn869776948 CALL NUMBER: Not available Request in: Jefferson or Adams Building Reading Rooms

Clinical evidence made easy LCCN: 2014451347 Type of material: Book Personal name: Harris, Michael, 1956 December 16- author. Main title: Clinical evidence made easy/M. Harris, General Practitioner and Visiting Senior Research Fellow in Bristol, UK, G. Taylor, Reader in Medical Statistics, University of Bath, UK, D. Jackson, Senior Research Fellow in Health Economics, University of Surrey, UK. Published/Produced: Banbury, U.K.: Scion, 2014. Description: xii, 212 pages; 24 cm. ISBN: 9781907904202 (pbk.) 1907904204 (pbk.) LC classification: R723.7 .H37 2014 Related names: Taylor, Gordon, 1970- author. Jackson, Daniel. Subjects: Evidence-based medicine. Evidence-based medicine--Methods. Evidence-Based Medicine. Evidence-based medicine. Notes: Includes index Dewey class no.: 610 NLM class no.: WA 950 H315c 2014 National bib agency no.: 016628441 Other system no.: (OCoLC)ocn868126317 Content type: text Media type: unmediated Carrier type: volume Shelf Location: FLM2015 027360 CALL NUMBER: R723.7 .H37 2014 OVERFLOWJ34 Request in: Jefferson or Adams Building Reading Rooms (FLM2)

Clinical therapeutics primer: link to the evidence for the ambulatory care pharmacist LCCN: 2012016800 Type of material: Book Main title: Clinical therapeutics primer: link to the evidence for the ambulatory care pharmacist/edited by Jennifer A. Reinhold, PharmD, BCPS, Assistant Professor, Philadelphia College of Pharmacy, University fo thye Sciences, Philadelphia, Pennsylvania, Grace Earl, PharmD, BCPS, Assistant Professor, Philadelphia College of Pharmacy, University of the Sciences, Philadelphia, Pennsylvania. Published/Created: Burlington, MA: Jones & Bartlett Learning, c2014. Description: xix, 444 p.; 26 cm. ISBN: 9781449687977 (pbk.: alk. paper) LC classification: RM300 .C57 2014 Related names: Reinhold, Jennifer A. Earl, Grace. Contents: Approach to the patient and the patient-centered care process -- Clinical trial evaluation and biostatistics primer -- Evidence-based medicine and the application to patient care -- Special populations and considerations: geriatric patients -- Special populations and considerations: pediatric patients -- Special populations and considerations: pregnancy and lactation -- Special populations and considerations: drug dosing in renal impairment -- Special populations and considerations: drug dosing in hepatic impairment -- Hypertension -- Diabetes -- Dyslipidemia -- Heart failure -- Anticoagulation -- Generalized anxiety disorder -- Major depressive disorder -- Chronic obstructive pulmonary disease and asthma -- Bone health -- Human immunodeficiency virus (HIV) -- Chronic pain. Subjects: Pharmaceutical Services. Ambulatory Care. Chronic Disease--drug therapy. Evidence-Based Medicine. Pharmacists. Notes: Includes bibliographical references and index. Dewey class no.: 362.12 NLM class no.: QV 737 Other system no.: (DNLM)101582966 CALL NUMBER: RM300 .C57 2014 Copy 1 Request in: Jefferson or Adams Building Reading Rooms

Clinical trials: design, conduct, and analysis LCCN: 2011036653 Type of material: Book Personal name: Meinert, Curtis L. Main title: Clinical trials: design, conduct, and analysis/Curtis L. Meinert. Edition: 2nd ed. Published/Created: New York: Oxford University Press, c2012. Description: xxxv, 665 p.: ill.; 26 cm. ISBN: 9780195387889 (hardback) 0195387880 (hardback) LC classification: R853.C55 M45 2012 Summary: "First published in 1986, this landmark text is the definitive guide to clinical trials, written by one of the leading experts in the field. This fully-updated second edition continues to be the most authoritative reference text on randomized clinical trials. It contains a wealth of practical information on the design, conduct, and analysis of both single center and multicenter trials. No other book on clinical trials offers as much detail on such issues as sample size calculation, stratification and randomization, data systems design, development of consent forms, publication policies, preparation of funding requests, and reporting procedures. While the basics of design, conduct, and analysis of clinical trials remain the same, there have been significant changes since the first edition of Clinical Trials was published two decades ago. In this new edition, the author discusses the refinements and improvements made to methods and procedures, changes in the policies and guidelines underlying trials, as well as requirements for registration of trials. He also discusses current practices for data sharing, for gender representation, for treatment effects monitoring, and for ethical standards of clinical trials. The importance of the randomized controlled trial has grown significantly over time and they are now the cornerstone of all evidence-based medicine. Still rich in tables, checklists, charts, and other resources for the trialist, the second edition of Clinical Trials is an indispensable reference for clinicians, biostaticians, epidemiologists, and anyone involved in the design and implementation of a clinical trial"--Provided by publisher. Subjects: Clinical trials. Clinical Trials as Topic Notes: Includes bibliographical references and index. Series: Monographs in epidemiology and biostatistics; 39 Monographs in epidemiology and biostatistics; v. 39. Dewey class no.: 616.0750724 NLM class no.: QV 771 M514c 2012 Other class no.: MED106000 MED028000 National bib agency no.: 015985877 Other system no.: (OCoLC)ocn756044508

Comparative effectiveness research: evidence, medicine, and policy LCCN: 2013006780 Type of material: Book Personal name: Ashton, Carol M. Main title: Comparative effectiveness research: evidence, medicine, and policy/Carol M. Ashton, Nelda P. Wray. Published/Created: Oxford; New York: Oxford University Press, c2013. Description: xiii, 290 p.; 25 cm. ISBN: 9780199968565 (hardback: alk. paper) 019996856X (hardback: alk. paper) 9780199969579 (e-book) 0199969574 (e-book) LC classification: RA440.87.U6 A84 2013 Related names: Wray, Nelda P. Contents: The generation of evidence in medicine: evaluating the benefits and harms of treatment -- The use of evidence: federal regulation of prescription drugs and medical devices -- The subversion of evidence: the Rosiglitazone story -- Operate first, evidence later: the special case of surgery -- Doctors and evidence: evidence-based medicine -- Comparative effective research: a new "silver bullet" for U.S. health care costs -- The legislative odyssey of comparative effectiveness research: birth in 2002 to the first federal mandate in 2003 -- 2005 to 2007: the health services research community stirs, the "B" word awakens policymakers, and the House CHAMP Act creates divisions -- 2008 to 2010: the Baucus-Conrad bills, the American Recovery and Reinvestment Act, and the Patient Protection and Affordable Care Act -- The scope, financing, and processes of federally-mandated comparative effectiveness research and why they matter -- Aligning clinical practice with best evidence of comparative effectiveness: payment policy for evidence-based medical care -- Dealing with uncertainty: payment policy for the generation of evidence as part of clinical practice. Subjects: Medical care--Research--United States--Evaluation. Evidence-based medicine--United States. Medical care, Cost of--Law and legislation--United States. Medical policy--United States. Comparative Effectiveness Research--history--United States. Health Care Costs--legislation & jurisprudence--United States. Comparative Effectiveness Research--legislation & jurisprudence--United States. Evidence-Based Medicine--United States. Government Regulation--United States. History, 21st Century--United States. Notes: Includes bibliographical references and index. Dewey class no.: 362.1072 NLM class no.: W 74 AA1 Other system no.: (DNLM)101602410 CALL NUMBER: RA440.87.U6 A84 2013 Copy 2 Request in: Jefferson or Adams Building Reading Rooms Shelf Location: FLM2013 005690 CALL NUMBER: RA440.87.U6 A84 2013 OVERFLOWA5S Request in: Jefferson or Adams Building Reading Rooms (FLM1)

Comprehensive systematic review for advanced nursing practice LCCN: 2011029339 Type of material: Book Personal name: Holly, Cheryl. Main title: Comprehensive systematic review for advanced nursing practice/Cheryl Holly, Susan W. Salmond, Marie K. Saimbert. Published/Created: New York: Springer Pub., c2012. Description: xxi, 336 p.: ill.; 26 cm. ISBN: 9780826117786 9780826117793 (e-book) LC classification: RT82.8 .H65 2012 Related names: Salmond, Susan Warner. Saimbert, Marie K. Contents: Systematic review as a basis for evidence-based practice/Susan Salmond and Cheryl Holly -- Steps in the systematic review process/Susan Salmond -- Planning and organizing a systematic review/Cheryl Holly -- Developing clinical questions/Marie K. Saimbert, Jenny Pierce, and Pam Hargwood -- Key principles for searching literature/Marie K. Saimbert -- Conducting searches: search resources and search techniques to maximize search efforts/Marie K. Saimbert ... [et al.] -- Critical appraisal/Susan Salmond -- Systematic review of experimental evidence: meta-analysis/Cheryl Holly -- Systematic review of observational evidence/Cheryl Holly -- Qualitative metasynthesis/Susan Salmond -- Systematic review of economic evidence/Cheryl Holly -- Systematic reviews and evidence-informed health care policy making/David Anthony Forrester, Rita Musanti, and Patricia Polansky -- Using systematic reviews at the point of care/Ronell Kirkley -- Future development of systematic reviews and evidence-based medicine/Jos Kleijnen. Subjects: Nurse practitioners. Advanced Practice Nursing. Review Literature as Topic. Evidence-Based Nursing--methods. Meta-Analysis as Topic. Notes: Includes bibliographical references and index. Dewey class no.: 610.73 NLM class no.: WY 128 Other system no.: (DNLM)101564287 CALL NUMBER: RT82.8 .H65 2012 Copy 1 Request in: Jefferson or Adams Building Reading Rooms

Controversies in neuro-oncology: best-evidence medicine for brain tumor surgery LCCN: 2013013422 Type of material: Book Main title: Controversies in neuro-oncology: best-evidence medicine for brain tumor surgery/[edited by] Alfredo Quiñones-Hinojosa, Shaan M. Raza. Published/Created: New York: Thieme, c2014. Description: xxiii, 495 p.: ill.; 29 cm. ISBN: 9781604067552 9781604067569 (eISBN) LC classification: RC280.B7 C58 2014 Related names: Quiñones-Hinojosa, Alfredo. Raza, Shaan M. Subjects: Brain Neoplasms--surgery. Brain Neoplasms--radiotherapy. Evidence-Based Medicine--methods. Neurosurgical Procedures. Radiosurgery--methods. Notes: Includes bibliographical references and index. Dewey class no.: 616.99/481 NLM class no.: WL 358 Other system no.: (DNLM)101605277 CALL NUMBER: RC280.B7 C58 2014 Copy 1 Request in: Jefferson or Adams Building Reading Rooms

Converting data into evidence: a statistics primer for the medical practioner LCCN: 2013942308 Type of material: Book Personal name: DeMaris, Alfred, 1946-, author. Main title: Converting data into evidence: a statistics primer for the medical practioner/Alfred DeMaris, Steven H. Selman. Published/Produced: New York: Springer, [2013] ©2013. Description: xv, 221 pages: illustrations; 24 cm ISBN: 9781461477914 (pbk.: alk. paper) 1461477913 (pbk.: alk. paper) 9781461477921 (ebk.) LC classification: R723.7 .D463 2013 Related names: Selman, Steven H., author. Subjects: Evidence-based medicine. Medical statistics. Notes: Includes bibliographical references (pages 211-214) and index. Dewey class no.: 610.72/7 NLM class no.: WB 102 Other system no.: (OCoLC)ocn859584792 Content type: text Media type: unmediated Carrier type: volume CALL NUMBER: R723.7 .D463 2013 Copy 2 Request in: Jefferson or Adams Building Reading Rooms Shelf Location: FLM2013 027573 CALL NUMBER: R723.7 .D463 2013 OVERFLOWA5S Request in: Jefferson or Adams Building Reading Rooms (FLM1)

Critical thinking skills for healthcare LCCN: 2015004044 Type of material: Book Personal name: McKendry, Stephanie, author. Main title: Critical thinking skills for healthcare/written by Stephanie McKendry. Published/Produced: Abingdon, Oxon; New York, NY: Routledge, 2015. Projected pub date: 1507 Description: p.; cm. ISBN: 9781138787513 (hbk) 9781138787520 (pbk.) LC classification: RC55 Contents: Taking a critical approach in everyday life -- Taking a critical approach at university -- Taking a critical approach to reading -- Building a rational and credible argument -- Taking a critical approach in assessments -- Taking a critical approach in literature reviews -- Taking a critical approach in dissertations -- Taking a critical approach in reflection and reflective assessments. Subjects: Clinical Competence. Evidence-Based Medicine. Decision Making. Health Knowledge, Attitudes, Practice. Problem-Based Learning. Thinking. Notes:

Includes bibliographical references and index. Dewey class no.: 616 NLM class no.: WB 102.5 Other system no.: (DNLM)101650689 Invalid ISBN: 9781315766409 (ebook) Content type: text Media type: unmediated Carrier type: volume

Current research in acupuncture LCCN: 2012939116 Type of material: Book Main title: Current research in acupuncture/Ying Xia, Guanghong Ding, Gen-Cheng Wu, editors. Published/Produced: New York: Springer, c2013 Description: xvi, 752 p.: ill. (some col.); 24 cm. ISBN: 9781461433569 (hardcover: alk. paper) 1461433568 (hardcover: alk. paper) 9781461433576 (ebook) 1461433576 (ebook) LC classification: RM184 .C87 2013 Related names: Xia, Ying, 1955- Ding, Guanghong. Wu, Gen-Cheng. Contents: Machine generated contents note: 1. Acupuncture Modulation of Neural Transmitters/Modulators/Ying Xia -- 2. Cellular Mechanisms in Acupuncture Points and Affected Sites/Quanbao Gu -- 3. Function of Collagen and Mast Cells in Acupuncture Points/Wei Yao -- 4. Functional Magnetic Resonance Imaging in Basic Acupuncture Research/Florian Beissner -- 5. Chemical and Physical Characteristics of Moxibustion/Xueyong Shen -- 6. Acupuncture Treatment of Epilepsy/Ying Xia -- 7. Acupuncture Treatment for Parkinson's Disease/Ying Xia -- 8. Can Acupuncture Treat Alzheimer's Disease and Other Neurodegenerative Disorders?/Ying Xia -- 9. Acupuncture Therapy for Vascular Cognitive Impairment/Zhiyan Sui -- 10. Acupuncture and Moxibustion for Antiaging/Huangan Wu -- 11. Development and Progression of Auricular Acupuncture as a Treatment for Anxiety and Pain/Shu-Ming Wang -- 12. Abdominal Acupuncture for Nerve Root Cervical Spondylosis/Yongjun Zheng. Note continued: 13. Electro-acupuncture Regulation of Central Monoamine Neurotransmitters in Ischaemia-Reperfusion/Dan Zhao -- 14. Protective Effect of Acupuncture on Myocardium/Yongjun Zheng -- 15. Acupuncture's Role in Cardiovascular Homeostasis/John C. Longhurst -- 16. Acupuncture in Polycystic Ovary Syndrome: Potential and Challenge/Boying Chen -- 17. Auricular Acupuncture for Pain and Inflammation/Yi Jie Zhan --

18. Glial-Neuronal Interactions in Electroacupuncture Analgesia/Yu-Qiu Zhang -- 19. Meridian-Viscera Correlationship/Lu He -- 20. Theory and Methodology of Evidence-Based Medicine in Acupuncture Research/Lei Lan -- 21. Chinese Medicine as a Model of System Biology: Diagnosis as the Foundation of Acupoint Selection/Henry Johannes Greten -- 22. Modernization of Acupuncture Using High-Tech Methods: Teleacupuncture Bridges Science and Practice/Gerhard Litscher. Subjects: Acupuncture. Acupuncture Therapy. Notes: Contents note continued: 23. Future Research in Acupuncture: Better Design and Analysis for Novel and Valid Findings/Ying Xia. Includes bibliographical references and index. Dewey class no.: 615.8/222 NLM class no.: 2012 I-205 WB 369 National bib agency no.: 101594754 016035692 Other system no.: (OCoLC)ocn773670659 Shelf Location: FLM2015 015328 CALL NUMBER: RM184 .C87 2013 OVERFLOWJ34 Request in: Jefferson or Adams Building Reading Rooms (FLM2)

Curriculum-based library instruction: from cultivating faculty relationships to assessment LCCN: 2014021093 Type of material: Book Main title: Curriculum-based library instruction: from cultivating faculty relationships to assessment/edited by Amy Blevins, Megan Inman. Published/Produced: Lanham: Rowman & Littlefield, [2014] Projected pub date: 1410 Description: pages cm. ISBN: 9781442239135 (cloth: alk. paper) 9781442231658 (pbk.: alk. paper) LC classification: Z711 .C875 2014 Related names: Blevins, Amy, 1981- editor. Inman, Megan, 1983- editor. Contents: Instructional roles for librarians/Jessica Cole -- Getting your foot in the door/Susan Kraat -- Introduction to learning theories/Rebecca S. Graves and Shelly R. McDavid -- Adult learning/Christine Andresen and Katy Kavanagh Webb -- Active learning/Barbara A. Gushrowski -- Introduction to instructional techniques/Rebecca S. Graves and Shelly R. McDavid -- Audience response systems/Emily Johnson -- Team based learning/Brandi Tuttle and Adrianne Leonardelli -- Lesson study in the nursing curriculum/Bryan S. Vogh, Hans Kishel, and Eric Jennings -- Online instruction/Megan B. Inman -- Face to face instruction/Michele Malloy and Sarah Cantrell -- Blended librarianship/Daniel P. Gall -- Incorporating self-assessment and peer assessment into library instructional practice/Stephan J. Macaluso -- What is evidence-based practice?/Connie Schardt -- Creating a curriculum based library instruction plan for medical students/Amy E. Blevins -- Librarians role in evidence-based medicine integration into the medical curriculum/Heather A. McEwen, Rienne Johnson, LuAnne M. Stockton, Janice M. Spalding, David M. Sperling, Lisa N. Weiss -- Reflections on involvement in a graduate nursing curriculum/Jennifer Deberg -- Strategies for building an information skills curriculum: the University of Michigan experience/Mark P. MacEachern and Whitney Townsend -- What is biomedical informatics?: an overview and case study/Carolyn Schubert -- What is information literacy?/April Cunningham and Allie Carr -- How to achieve information literacy integration/Allie Carr and April Cunningham -- A curricular approach to information literacy instruction in sociology: a case study/Adam T. Beauchamp -- Evolution of an undergraduate business information literacy class: a case study/Kimberly Bloedel -- The expanding role of information literacy in the freshman writing program at Saint Louis University: a case study/Jamie L. Emery. Subjects: Library orientation. Library orientation for medical students. Information literacy--Study and teaching. Academic libraries--Relations with faculty and curriculum. Medical librarians. Notes: Includes bibliographical references and index. Series: Medical Library Association books Dewey class no.: 025.5/6 Invalid ISBN: 9781442231665 (ebook) Content type: text Media type: unmediated Carrier type: volume

Decision making in emergency critical care: an evidence-based handbook LCCN: 2014004152 Type of material: Book Main title: Decision making in emergency critical care: an evidence-based handbook/editor, John E. Arbo, MD, Assistant Professor of Emergency Medicine and Critical Care Medicine, New York-Presbyterian Hospital/Weill Cronell Medical Center, New York, New York; associate editors, Stephen J. Ruoss, MD, Professor of Pulmonary and Critical Care Medicine, Stanford

University Medical Center, Stanford, California, Geoffrey K. Lighthall, MD, Associate Professor of Anesthesia and Crtical Care Medicine, Stanford University Medical Center, Stanford, California, Michael P. Jones, MD, Assistant Professor of Emergency Medicine, Associate Program Director-Jacobi/Montefiore Emergency Medicine Residency Program, Albert Einstein College of Medicine, New York, New York; special editor: neurology section: Joshua Stillman, MD, MPH, Assistant Professor of Medicine, Emergency Medicine Director of the Stroke Center at New York-Presbyterian Hospital/Columbia University Medical Center, New York, New York. Published/Produced: Philadelphia: Wolters Kluwer, [2015] ©2015 Description: xxi, 810 pages: illustrations; 23 cm Links: Table of contents only http://www.loc.gov/catdir/enhancements/fy1503/2014004152-t.html Contributor biographical information http://www.loc.gov/catdir/enhancements/fy1503/2014004152-b.html Publisher description http://www.loc.gov/catdir/enhancements/fy1503/2014004152-d.html ISBN: 9781451186895 1451186894 LC classification: RC86.7 .D443 2015 Related names: Arbo, John E., editor of compilation. Ruoss, Stephen, editor of compilation. Lighthall, Geoffrey K., editor of compilation. Jones, Michael P., 1981- editor of compilation. Stillman, Joshua, editor of compilation. Subjects: Critical Care. Decision Making. Emergency Service, Hospital. Emergency Treatment--methods. Evidence-Based Medicine. Notes: Includes bibliographical references. Dewey class no.: 616.02/8 NLM class no.: WX 218 Other system no.: (DNLM)101624895 Content type: text Media type: unmediated Carrier type: volume Shelf Location: FLM2015 003730 CALL NUMBER: RC86.7 .D443 2015 OVERFLOWJ34 Request in: Jefferson or Adams Building Reading Rooms (FLM2)

Decision making in health and medicine: integrating evidence and values LCCN: 2014000260 Type of material: Book Personal name: Hunink, M. G. Myriam, author. Main title: Decision making in health and medicine: integrating evidence and values/M.G. Myriam Hunink, Milton C. Weinstein, Eve Wittenberg, Michael F. Drummond, Joseph S. Pliskin, John B. Wong, Paul P. Glasziou.

Edition: Second edition. Published/Produced: Cambridge, United Kingdom: Cambridge University Press, 2014. Description: xxi, 424 pages: illustrations; 24 cm. ISBN: 9781107690479 (pbk.) 1107690471 (pbk.) LC classification: R723.5 .H86 2014 Contents: Elements of decision making in health care -- Managing uncertainty -- Choosing the best treatment -- Valuing outcomes -- Interpreting diagnostic information -- Deciding when to test -- Multiple test results -- Finding and summarizing the evidence -- Constrained resources -- Recurring events -- Estimation, calibration, and validation -- Heterogeneity and uncertainty -- Psychology of judgment and choice. Subjects: Medicine--Decision making. Medical care--Decision making. Evidence-based medicine. Values. Decision Making. Delivery of Health Care. Decision Support Techniques. Evidence-Based Medicine. Uncertainty. Notes: Preceded by Decision making in health and medicine: integrating evidence and values/M.G. Myriam Hunink ... [et al.]. 2001. Includes bibliographical references and index. Series: Cambridge medicine Dewey class no.: 610 NLM class no.: W 84.1 Other system no.: (DNLM)101623172 Content type: text Media type: unmediated Carrier type: volume CALL NUMBER: R723.5 .H86 2014 Copy 1 Request in: Jefferson or Adams Building Reading Rooms

Delivering Affordable Cancer Care in the 21st Century: workshop Summary: LCCN: 2013444474 Type of material: Book Meeting name Delivering Affordable Cancer Care in the 21st Century (Workshop) (2012: Washington, D.C.), author. Main title: Delivering Affordable Cancer Care in the 21st Century: workshop summary/Erin Balogh, Margie Patlak, and Sharyl J. Nass, rapporteurs; National Cancer Policy Forum, Board on Health Care Services, Institute of Medicine of the National Academies. Published/Produced: Washington, D.C.: National Academies Press, [2013] ©2013 Description: xiv, 80 pages: illustrations (some color), color map; 24 cm ISBN: 9780309269445 (pbk.) 030926944X (pbk.) LC classification: RC270.8 .D45 2013 Related names: Balogh, Erin. Patlak, Margie. Nass, Sharyl J. National Cancer Policy Forum (U.S.), sponsoring body.

Institute of Medicine (U.S.). Board on Health Care Services, issuing body. Summary: "Rising health care costs are a central fiscal challenge confronting the United States. National spending on health care currently accounts for 18 percent of gross domestic product (GDP), but is anticipated to increase to 25 percent of GDP by 2037. The Bipartisan Policy Center argues that "this rapid growth in health expenditures creates an unsustainable burden on America's economy, with far-reaching consequences". These consequences include crowding out many national priorities, including investments in education, infrastructure, and research; stagnation of employee wages; and decreased international competitiveness. In spite of health care costs that far exceed those of other countries, health outcomes in the United States are not considerably better. With the goal of ensuring that patients have access to high-quality, affordable cancer care, the Institute of Medicine's (IOM's) National Cancer Policy Forum convened a public workshop, Delivering Affordable Cancer Care in the 21st Century, October 8-9, 2012, in Washington, DC. Delivering Affordable Cancer Care in the 21st Century summarizes the workshop"-- Publisher's description. Contents: Introduction -- A financial crisis in health care -- Drivers of health care costs -- Cancer care costs -- Financial burden on patients with cancer -- Questionable value -- Current challenges -- Inappropriate incentives -- Unrealistic expectations -- Overuse and misuse of interventions -- Variable care, lack of best practices, and an inadequate evidence base -- Legal and regulatory issues -- Assessing value -- Possible solutions -- Patient and clinician communication and education -- Best practices in cancer care -- Evidence base for clinical practice and reimbursement -- Financial incentives aligned with affordable, high-quality cancer care -- Delivery system and reimbursement changes -- Wrap up. Subjects: Cancer--Treatment--Congresses. Medical care, Cost of--Congresses. Medical care--Finance--Congresses. Health Care Costs--United States--Congresses. Neoplasms--therapy--United States--Congresses. Evidence-Based Medicine--United States--Congresses. Health Services--economics--United States--Congresses. Neoplasms--

economics--United States--Congresses. Practice Guidelines as Topic--United States--Congresses. Notes: Includes bibliographical references (pages 67-74). Dewey class no.: 616.99406 NLM class no.: 2013 G-559 QZ 266 National bib agency no.: 101613693 Other system no.: (OCoLC)ocn830351870 Content type: text Media type: unmediated Carrier type: volume CALL NUMBER: RC270.8 .D45 2013 Copy 2 Request in: Jefferson or Adams Building Reading Rooms Shelf Location: FLM2014 041461 CALL NUMBER: RC270.8 .D45 2013 OVERFLOWA5S Request in: Jefferson or Adams Building Reading Rooms (FLM1)

Developing Evidence-Based Generalist Practice Skills LCCN: 2012026666 Type of material: Book Main title: Developing Evidence-Based Generalist Practice Skills/edited by Bruce A. Thyer, Catherine N. Dulmus, Karen M. Sowers. Published/Produced: Hoboken, New Jersey: John Wiley & Sons, Inc., [2013] Description: xviii, 238 pages; 25 cm ISBN: 9781118176962 (pbk.) LC classification: R723.7 .D484 2013 Related names: Thyer, Bruce A., editor of compilation. Dulmus, Catherine N., editor of compilation. Sowers, Karen M. (Karen Marlaine), editor of compilation. Contents: Evidence-informed practice/Eileen Gambrill -- Trauma-informed practice/Nancy J. Smyth & Laura Greyber -- Interviewing skills/Francis J. Turner -- Problem identification, contracting, and case planning/Sophia F. Dziegielewski -- Case management/Valerie Holton and Joseph Walsh -- Advocacy/Malabika Misty Das, Cheryl Hiu-Kwan Chui, and Cecilia Lai-Wan Chan -- Crisis intervention/Kenneth R. Yeager, Albert R. Roberts, and Wendy Grainger -- Practice evaluation/Bruce A. Thyer -- Termination, stabilization, and continuity of care/Samuel A. MacMaster and Sara Sanders. Subjects: Evidence-based medicine. Physicians (General practice) Notes: Includes bibliographical references and indexes. Dewey class no.: 610.69/5 Invalid ISBN: 9781118433775 (ebk.) 9781118421178 (ebk.) 9781118419328 (ebk.) Content type: text Media type: unmediated Carrier type: volume CALL NUMBER: R723.7 .D484 2013 Copy 1 Request in:

Jefferson or Adams Building Reading Rooms

Dissemination and implementation of evidence-based psychological interventions LCCN: 2011031967 Type of material: Book Main title: Dissemination and implementation of evidence-based psychological interventions/edited by R. Kathryn McHugh and David H. Barlow. Published/Created: Oxford: Oxford University Press, c2012. Description: xiv, 274 p.; 25 cm. ISBN: 9780195389050 (alk. paper) LC classification: RC455.2.E94 D57 2012 Related names: McHugh, R. Kathryn (Rebecca Kathryn) Barlow, David H. Contents: The reach of evidence-based psychological interventions/R. Kathryn McHugh and David H. Barlow -- The science of dissemination and implementation/Sonja K. Schoenwald, R. Kathryn McHugh, and David H. Barlow -- Training in evidence-based psychological interventions/R. Kathryn McHugh and David H. Barlow -- The English improving access to psychological therapies (IAPT) program: history and progress/David M. Clark -- Implementation of evidence-based psychological treatments in the Veterans Health Administration/Josef I. Ruzek, Bradley E. Karlin, and Antonette Zeiss -- Development and application of the NCCTS learning collaborative model for the implementation of evidence-based child trauma treatment/Lori Ebert ... [et al.] -- Evidence-based practice and autism: building systemic capacity based on the National Standards Project/Susan M. Wilczynski, Dennis Russo, and Walter P. Christian -- The dissemination of evidence-based practices by federal and state mental health agencies/Jeanne C. Rivard ... [et al.] -- Sustaining Hawaii's evidence-based service system in children's mental health/Brad J. Nakamura, Charmaine K. Higa-McMillan, and Bruce F. Chorpita -- Dissemination of dialectical behavior therapy: an intensive training model/Sara J. Landes and Marsha M. Linehan -- Enhancing dissemination outcomes through a population-based approach to parenting intervention/Matthew R. Sanders and Rachel Calam -- The transport and diffusion of multisystemic therapy/Sonja K. Schoenwald -- Dissemination and implementation of evidence-based psychological interventions: current status and future directions/R. Kathryn McHugh & David H. Barlow. Subjects: Mental Disorders--prevention & control. Mental Disorders--therapy. Evidence-Based Medicine--methods. Information Dissemination--methods. Psychotherapy--methods. Notes: Includes bibliographical references and index. Dewey class no.: 616.89 NLM class no.: WM 400 Other system no.: (DNLM)101565983 Shelf Location: FLM2013 012589 CALL NUMBER: RC455.2.E94 D57 2012 OVERFLOWA5S Request in: Jefferson or Adams Building Reading Rooms (FLM1)

Ending medical reversal: improving outcomes, saving lives LCCN: 2014049513 Type of material: Book Personal name: Prasad, Vinayak K., 1982-, author. Main title: Ending medical reversal: improving outcomes, saving lives/Vinayak K. Prasad and Adam S. Cifu. Published/Produced: Baltimore: Johns Hopkins University Press, 2015. Projected pub date: 1510 Description: p.; cm. ISBN: 9781421417721 (hardcover: alk. paper) 1421417723 (hardcover: alk. paper) LC classification: R733 Related names: Cifu, Adam S., author. Contents: What is medical reversal? -- Subjective outcomes: why feeling better is often misleading -- Surrogate outcomes -- Screening tests -- System failure -- Finding flawed therapies on our own -- The frequency of medical reversal -- The harms of medical reversal: today's patients, tomorrow's patients and the healthcare field -- A primer in evidence based medicine: what is evidence in medicine? -- What really got you better: when evidence gets complicated -- Scientific progress, revolution, and medical reversal -- Sources of flawed data -- Why are we so attracted to flawed therapies? -- Medical education: a very good place to start -- Academic medicine -- Reforming the system: the burden of proof and nudging our way past reversal -- How not to become a victim of reversal -- Beyond dogma: when randomized trials are unnecessary. Subjects: Delivery of Health Care. Treatment Outcome. Clinical Trials as Topic. Evidence-Based Medicine. Therapeutics--trends. Form/Genre: Popular Works. Notes: Includes bibliographical references and index. Dewey class no.: 615.5 NLM class no.: W 84.41 Other system no.: (DNLM)101648973 Invalid ISBN: 9781421417738 (electronic) 1421417731 (electronic) Content type: text Media type: unmediated Carrier type: volume

Essential evidence-based psychopharmacology LCCN: 2011053165 Type of material: Book Main title: Essential evidence-based psychopharmacology/edited by Dan J. Stein, Bernard Lerer, Stephen M. Stahl. Edition: 2nd ed. Published/Created: Cambridge; New York: Cambridge University Press, 2012. Description: viii, 325 p.: ill.; 24 cm. ISBN: 9781107007956 (hardback) 110700795X (hardback) 9781107400108 (pbk.) 1107400104 (pbk.) LC classification: RC483 .E95 2012 Related titles: Evidence-based pharmacology. Related names: Stein, Dan J. Lerer, Bernard. Stahl, Stephen M., 1951- Subjects: Mental illness--Chemotherapy. Psychotropic drugs. Psychopharmacology. Evidence-based medicine. Notes: Rev. ed. of: Evidence-based phamacology. Includes bibliographical references and index. Dewey class no.: 616.89/18 CALL NUMBER: RC483 .E95 2012 Copy 1 Request in: Jefferson or Adams Building Reading Rooms

Essential values-based practice: clinical stories linking science with people LCCN: 2012405392 Type of material: Book Personal name: Fulford, K. W. M. Main title: Essential values-based practice: clinical stories linking science with people/by K.W.M. (Bill) Fulford, Ed Peile, Heidi Carroll. Published/Created: Cambridge; New York: Cambridge University Press, 2012. Description: xv, 215 p.: ill.; 25 cm. ISBN: 9780521530255 (pbk.) 0521530253 (pbk.) LC classification: R728 .F83 2012 Related names: Peile, Ed. Carroll, Heidi. Contents: Foreword, from a patient perspective -- Foreword, from a clinician perspective -- A bold claim to start this book -- Prologue: linking science with people -- Values, individuals and an overview of values-based practice: introduction to 'it's my back, doctor!' (episode 1): values in clinical decision making -- 'It's my back, Doctor!' (episode 2): applying the tools already in the clinical toolbox for working with values to individuals -- An outline of values-based practice: its point, premise and ten-part process -- The clinical skills for values-based practice: introduction to recovery in schizophrenia: a values wake-up call -- Teenage acne: widening our values horizons -- A smoking enigma: getting (and not getting) the knowledge -- Diabetic control and controllers: nothing without communication -- Relationships in values-based practice: introduction to 'best' in breast cancer: clinician values and person-centred care -- Risks in safeguarding children: team values as well as skills -- Science and values-based practice: introduction to the reluctant hypertensive: think evidence, think values too! -- Unexplainable abdominal pain: think values, think evidence too! -- Elective fertility: think high-tech, think evidence and values! -- Bringing it all together: introduction to a good (enough) death: dissensus in end of life care -- 'It's my back, Doctor!' (episode 3) -- Postscript: the small change of care -- A bold claim to end this book. Subjects: Medicine--Practice. Clinical medicine. Medical ethics. Physician and patient. Delivery of Health Care--ethics. Evidence-Based Medicine. Physician-Patient Relations. Social Values. Notes: Includes bibliographical references and index. Series: Cambridge medicine Cambridge medicine. Dewey class no.: 610.6 NLM class no.: 2012 E-223 W 84.1 National bib no.: GBB1D9327 National bib agency no.: 101585200 015986182 Other system no.: (OCoLC)ocn768071778 CALL NUMBER: R728 .F83 2012 Copy 1 Request in: Jefferson or Adams Building Reading Rooms CALL NUMBER: R728 .F83 2012 LANDOVR Copy 2 Request in: Jefferson or Adams Building Reading Rooms - STORED OFFSITE

Ethical oversight of learning health care systems. LCCN: 2012554504 Type of material: Book Main title: Ethical oversight of learning health care systems. Published/Created: [Malden, Mass.]: Wiley-Blackwell, [2013] Description: 44 p.: ill.; 28 cm. LC classification: R723.7 .E83 2013 Related names: Solomon, Mildred Z. Bonham, Ann. Hastings Center. Contents: Ethical oversight of research on patient health care/Mildred Z. Solomon and Ann Bonham -- The research-treatment distinction: a problematic approach for determining which activities should have ethical oversight/Nancy E. Klass ... [et al.] -- An ethics framework for a learning health care system: a departure from traditional research ethics and clinical ethics/Ruth R. Fadden ... [et al.] -- A prescription for ethical learning/Emily A. Largent, Franklin G. Miller, and Steven Joffe -- The unbelievable rightness of being in clinical trials/Jerry Menikoff -- Making the transition to a learning health care system/Christine Grady and David Wendler -- Ethical oversight: serving the best interests of patients/Joe V. Selby and Harlan M. Krumholz -- Evaluation as part of operations: reconciling the common rule and continuous improvement/Richard Platt, Claudia Grossman, and Harry P. Selker -- Reform within the common rule?/Tom Puglisi -- Advances in the research enterprise/Joel Kupersmith. Subjects: Evidence-based medicine--Moral and ethical aspects. Medical ethics. Notes: Cover title. "Guest editors ... were Mildred Z. Solomon ... and Ann Bonham"--P. [2] of cover. Includes bibliographical references. Series: An HCR special report; v.43, issue s1 Hastings Center special report; v.43, issue s1. Dewey class no.: 174.2 Other system no.: (OCoLC)ocn824695412 CALL NUMBER: R723.7 .E83 2013 LANDOVR Copy 2 Request in: Jefferson or Adams Building Reading Rooms - STORED OFFSITE Shelf Location: FLM2014 023405 CALL NUMBER: R723.7 .E83 2013 OVERFLOWA5S Request in: Jefferson or Adams Building Reading Rooms (FLM1)

Evidence and skills for normal labour and birth: guide for midwives LCCN: 2011021491 Type of material: Book Personal name: Walsh, Denis, 1955- Main title: Evidence and skills for normal labour and birth: guide for midwives/Denis Walsh. Edition: 2nd ed. Published/Created: Abingdon, Oxon: Routledge, 2012. Description: xviii, 206 p.: ill.; 25 cm. ISBN: 9780415577311 (hbk) 9780415577328 (pbk) 9780203357361 (ebk) LC classification: RG651 .W35 2012 Related names: Walsh, Denis, 1955- Evidence-based care for normal labour and birth. Summary: "Evidence-based care is a well established principle in contemporary healthcare and a worldwide health care movement. However, despite the emphasis on promoting evidence-based or effective care without the unnecessary use of technologies and drugs, intervention rates in childbirth continue to rise rapidly. This new edition emphasises the importance of translating evidence into skilful practice. It updates the evidence around what works best for normal birth, aspects of which still remain hidden and ignored by some maternity care professionals. Beginning with the decision about where to have a baby, through all the phases of labour to the immediate post-birth period, it systematically details research and other evidence sources that endorse a low intervention approach. The second edition: - has been expanded with new chapters on Preparation for Childbirth and Waterbirth - highlights where the evidence is compelling - discusses its application where women question its relevance to them and where the practitioner's expertise leads them to challenge it - gives background and context before discussing the research to date - includes questions for reflection, skills sections and practice recommendations generated from the evidence. Using evidence drawn from a variety of sources, Evidence and Skills for Normal Labour and Birth critiques institutionalised, scientifically managed birth and endorses a more humane midwifery-led model. Packed with up-to-date and relevant information, this text will help all students, practising midwives and doulas keep abreast of the evidence surrounding normal birth and ensure their practice takes full advantage of it"-- Provided by publisher. Subjects: Labor (Obstetrics) Childbirth. Evidence-based medicine. Natural Childbirth--nursing. Evidence-Based Medicine. Midwifery. Notes: Rev. ed. of: Evidence-based care for normal labour and birth/Denis Walsh. 2007. Includes bibliographical references and index. Dewey class no.: 618.4 NLM class no.: WQ 152 Other system no.: (DNLM)101561098 CALL NUMBER: RG651 .W35 2012 Copy 1 Request in: Jefferson or Adams Building Reading Rooms

Evidence based physical therapy LCCN: 2012002237 Type of material: Book Personal name: Fetters, Linda, 1948- Main title: Evidence based physical therapy/Linda Fetters, Julie Tilson. Published/Created: Philadelphia: F.A. Davis Co., c2012. Description: xviii, 182 p.: ill.; 28 cm. ISBN: 9780803617162 (pbk.: alk. paper) LC classification: RM701 .F48 2012 Related names: Tilson, Julie. Subjects: Physical Therapy Modalities. Evidence-Based Medicine. Notes: Includes bibliographical references and index. Dewey class no.: 615.8/2 NLM class no.: WB 460 Other system no.: (DNLM)101576525 CALL NUMBER: RM701 .F48 2012 Copy 1 Request in: Jefferson or Adams Building Reading Rooms

Evidence based treatments for eating disorders: children, adolescents and adults LCCN: 2014932381 Type of material: Book Main title: Evidence based treatments for eating disorders: children, adolescents and adults/Ida F. Dancyger, PH.D. and Victor M. Fornari, M.D., editors. Edition: Second edition. Published/Produced: New York: Nova Biomedical, [2014] Description: xxvii, 582 pages: illustrations; 26 cm. ISBN: 9781631174001 (hardcover) LC classification: RC552.E18 E95 2014 Related names: Dancyger, Ida F., editor. Fornari, Victor M., editor. Subjects: Eating disorders. Evidence-based medicine. Notes: Includes bibliographical references and index. Series: Eating disorders in the 21st century Dewey class no.: 616.85/26 Content type: text Media type: unmediated Carrier type: volume Shelf Location: FLM2014 166852 CALL NUMBER: RC552.E18 E95 2014 OVERFLOWA5S Request in: Jefferson or Adams Building Reading Rooms (FLM1)

Evidence into practice: integrating judgment, values, and research LCCN: 2012033718 Type of material: Book Personal name: Hack, Laurita Mary. Main title: Evidence into practice: integrating judgment, values, and research/Laurita M. Hack, Jan Gwyer. Published/Created: Philadelphia: F.A. Davis Co., c2013. Description: xix, 364 p.: ill.; 26 cm. ISBN: 9780803618084 (pbk.: alk. paper) LC classification: RM708 .H37 2013 Related names: Gwyer, Jan. Contents: The language of practice -- How physical therapists make clinical decisions -- Mistakes and errors: when clinical decisions go wrong -- Biases in clinical reasoning: most of my patients are helped by this treatment/John C. Hershey -- Clinical decision making tools -- Bridging the differences of diversity: communicating in the borderlands/Suzanne P. Gordon -- The patient interview/Jack Coulehan, Marian R. Block -- Learning about patients' perspectives: qualitative research/Kim Nixon-Cave -- The health care system and patient circumstances/Michael P. Johnson -- Asking clinical questions -- Finding the evidence/Connie Schardt -- Elements of good research practice -- The individual study as a source of evidence -- Synopses of studies -- Synthesis of studies through systematic reviews and meta-analyses/Alison Bailey Hallam -- Summaries and systems -- Translating evidence into practice -- Documentation as evidence/Kristin von Nieda -- Quality improvement in action/Christopher G. Bise, Anthony DeLitto. Subjects: Physical Therapy Modalities. Biomedical Research. Decision Making. Evidence-Based Medicine. Professional-Patient Relations. Notes: Includes bibliographical references. Dewey class no.: 610.72/4 NLM class no.: WB 460 Other system no.: (DNLM)101590707 Shelf Location: FLM2014 020476 CALL NUMBER: RM708 .H37 2013 OVERFLOWA5S Request in: Jefferson or Adams Building Reading Rooms (FLM1)

Evidence synthesis for decision making in healthcare LCCN: 2011051684 Type of material: Book Main title: Evidence synthesis for decision making in healthcare/Nicky J. Welton ... [et al.]. Published/Created: Chichester, West Sussex: John Wiley & Sons, 2012. Projected pub date: 1208 Description: p.; cm. ISBN: 9780470061091 (cloth) Related names: Welton, Nicky J. Contents: Introduction -- Bayesian methods and winBUGS -- Introduction to decision models -- Meta-analysis using Bayesian methods -- Exploring between study heterogeneity -- Model critique and evidence consistency in random effects meta-analysis -- Evidence synthesis in a decision modelling framework -- Multi-parameter evidence synthesis in epidemiological models -- Mixed treatment comparisons -- Markov models -- Generalised evidence synthesis -- Expected value of information for research prioritisation and study design. Subjects: Decision Support Techniques. Statistics as Topic. Evidence-Based Medicine--economics. Models, Statistical. Notes: Includes bibliographical references and index. Dewey class no.: 362.1068/4 NLM class no.: WB 102.5 Other system no.: (DNLM)101575193 CALL NUMBER: Not available Request in: Jefferson or Adams Building Reading Rooms

Evidence-based dermatology LCCN: 2013049542 Type of material: Book Uniform title: Evidence-based dermatology (Williams)

Main title: Evidence-based dermatology/edited by Hywel C. Williams; associate editors, Michael Bigby [and six others]. Edition: Third edition. Published/Produced: Chichester, West Sussex: John Wiley & Sons, Ltd, 2014. Projected pub date: 1405 Description: p.; cm. ISBN: 9781118357675 (cloth) LC classification: RL71 Related names: Williams, Hywel C., editor of compilation. Bigby, Michael E., editor of compilation. Subjects: Skin Diseases. Evidence-Based Medicine. Notes: Includes bibliographical references and index. Additional formats: Online version: Third edition. Chichester, West Sussex: John Wiley & Sons, Ltd, 2014 9781118357637 (DLC) 2013051087 Dewey class no.: 616.5 NLM class no.: WR 140 Other system no.: (DNLM)101622083 Content type: text Media type: unmediated Carrier type: volume

Evidence-based endocrinology LCCN: 2011051079 Type of material: Book Main title: Evidence-based endocrinology/editors, Pauline M. Camacho, MD, FACE, Associate Professor of Medicine, Division of Endocrinology and Metabolism, Director, Loyola University Osteoporosis and Metabolic Bone Disease Center, Department of Medicine, Loyola University Chicago Stritch School of Medicine, Chicago, Illinois, Hossein Gharib, MD, MACP, MACE, Professor of Medicine, Division of Endocrinology, Metabolism, and Nutrition, Department of Medicine, Mayo Clinic College of Medicine, Rochester, Minnesota, Past President, American Associate of Clinical Endocrinologists, Glen W. Sizemore, MD, FACE, Emeritus Professor of Medicine, Loyola University of Chicago Stritch School of Medicine, Chicago, Illinois. Edition: Third edition. Published/Produced: Philadelphia: Wolters Kluwer Health/Lippincott Williams & Wilkins Health, [2012] Description: xxii, 412 pages: illustrations; 21 cm Links: Publisher description http://www.loc.gov/catdir/enhancements/fy1205/2011051079-d.html ISBN: 9781451110913 (pbk.) 145111091X (pbk.) LC classification: RC649 .E95 2012 Related names: Camacho, Pauline M. Gharib, Hossein, 1940- Sizemore, Glen W. Contents: Hypothalamic-pituitary disease/Gerald Charnogursky ... [et al.] --

Thyroid disorders/M. Regina Castro and Hossein Gharib -- Adrenal disorders/Dana Erickson and Steven A. De Jong -- Metabolic bone disorders/Alaleh Mazhari, Zeina Habib, and Pauline Camacho -- Reproductive disorders/Neil Goodman and Rhoda H. Cobin -- Diabetes mellitus/Haitham S. Abu-Lebdeh and Gregg D. Simonson -- Lipid disorders/Francis Q. Almeda and Susan DeLange -- Obesity and nutrition/Jeffrey I. Mechanick and Elise M. Brett -- Multiple endocrine neoplasia/Glen Sizemore and Norma Lopez -- Carcinoid tumors/Nathan J. O'Dorisio, Thomas M. O'Dorisio, and M. Sue O'Dorisio -- Paraneoplastic syndromes/Subhash Kukreja -- Genetics/Peter Kopp. Subjects: Endocrine System Diseases--Handbooks. Endocrine System Diseases--Review. Cost-Benefit Analysis--methods--Handbooks. Cost-Benefit Analysis--methods--Review. Evidence-Based Medicine--methods--Handbooks. Evidence-Based Medicine--methods--Review. Treatment Outcome--Handbooks. Treatment Outcome--Review. Notes: Includes bibliographical references and index. Dewey class no.: 616.4 NLM class no.: WK 39 Other system no.: (DNLM)101574387 Content type: text Media type: unmediated Carrier type: volume CALL NUMBER: RC649 .E95 2012 Copy 1 Request in: Jefferson or Adams Building Reading Rooms CALL NUMBER: RC649 .E95 2012 LANDOVR Copy 2 Request in: Jefferson or Adams Building Reading Rooms - STORED OFFSITE

Evidence-based healthcare in context: critical social science perspectives LCCN: 2011040154 Type of material: Book Personal name: Broom, Alex. Main title: Evidence-based healthcare in context: critical social science perspectives/by Alex Broom and Jon Adams. Published/Created: Farnham, Surrey, UK; Burlington, VT: Ashgate Pub. Co., c2012. Description: xi, 195 p.; 24 cm. ISBN: 9780754679813 (hardback: alk. paper) LC classification: R723.7 .B76 2012 Variant title: Evidence based health care in context Related names: Adams, Jon, 1971- Subjects: Evidence-based medicine. Social medicine. Notes: Includes bibliographical references and index. Dewey class no.: 362.1 CALL NUMBER: R723.7 .B76 2012

Copy 1 Request in: Jefferson or Adams Building Reading Rooms CALL NUMBER: R723.7 .B76 2012 Copy 2 Request in: Jefferson or Adams Building Reading Rooms

Evidence-based management of diabetes LCCN: 2012538075 Type of material: Book Main title: Evidence-based management of diabetes/[edited by] Jiten Vora, John Buse. Edition: 1st ed. Published/Created: Harley, UK: tfm Pub., c2012. Description: xiv, 506 p.: ill. (some col.); 25 cm. ISBN: 9781903378786 1903378788 LC classification: RC660 .E94 2012 Related names: Vora, Jiten. Buse, John B. Subjects: Diabetes--Treatment. Evidence-based medicine. Diabetes Mellitus--therapy. Evidence-Based Medicine. Notes: Includes bibliographical references and index. Dewey class no.: 616.4/62 NLM class no.: 2012 I-436 WK 815 National bib agency no.: 101595489 Other system no.: (OCoLC)ocn816100673 CALL NUMBER: RC660 .E94 2012 Copy 1 Request in: Jefferson or Adams Building Reading Rooms

Evidence-based management of low back pain LCCN: 2011499245 Type of material: Book Main title: Evidence-based management of low back pain/editors, Simon Dagenais, Scott Haldeman. Published/Created: St Louis, Mo.: Elsevier Mosby, c2012. Description: xviii, 478 p.: ill.; 29 cm. ISBN: 9780323072939 0323072933 LC classification: RD771.B217 E95 2012 Variant title: Low back pain Related names: Dagenais, Simon. Haldeman, Scott. Contents: Introduction -- [Patient] Education -- Exercise -- Medication -- Physical modalities -- Manual therapies -- Complementary and alternative medical therapies -- Behavioral therapies -- Injection therapies - Minimally invasive therapies -- Surgical therapies. -- Conclusion -- Answers to review questions. Subjects: Backache--Treatment. Low Back Pain--therapy. Evidence-Based Medicine. Notes: Includes bibliographical references and index. Dewey class no.: 617.5/64 NLM class no.: 2011 D-483 WE 755 National bib agency no.: 101557780 Other system no.: (OCoLC)ocn659752013 CALL NUMBER: RD771.B217 E95 2012 Copy 1 Request in: Jefferson or Adams Building Reading Rooms CALL NUMBER: RD771.B217 E95

2012 Copy 2 Request in: Jefferson or Adams Building Reading Rooms

Evidence-based medicine: reading and writing medical papers LCCN: 2012047788 Type of material: Book Personal name: Kaura, Amit. Main title: Evidence-based medicine: reading and writing medical papers/Amit Kaura. Published/Created: Edinburgh: Mosby/Elsevier, 2013. Projected pub date: 1308 Description: p.; cm. ISBN: 9780723437352 Contents: Evidence-based medicine -- Handling data -- Investigating hypotheses -- Systematic review and meta-analysis -- Research design -- Randomized controlled trials -- Cohort studies -- Case-control studies -- Measures of disease occurrence and cross-sectional studies -- Ecological studies -- Case report and case series -- Qualitative research -- Confounding -- Screening, diagnosis and prognosis -- Statistical techniques -- Clinical audit -- Quality improvement -- Economic evaluation -- Critical appraisal checklists -- Crash course in statistical formulae -- Careers in academic medicine. Subjects: Evidence-Based Medicine. Biomedical Research. Data Collection. Reading. Writing. Notes: Includes index. Series: Crash course Crash course. Dewey class no.: 610.72 NLM class no.: WB 102.5 Other system no.: (DNLM)101596895

Evidence-based neonatal infections LCCN: 2013026696 Type of material: Book Personal name: Isaacs, David, 1950- author. Main title: Evidence-based neonatal infections/David Isaacs. Published/Produced: Chichester, West Sussex, UK: John Wiley & Sons Inc., 2014 Projected pub date: 1405 Description: p.; cm. ISBN: 9780470654606 (pbk.) LC classification: RJ254 Contents: How to search for evidence -- Epidemiology -- Clinical manifestations -- Laboratory tests -- Rational antibiotic use -- Adjunctive treatment -- Bacterial meningitis -- Respiratory tract infections -- Osteomyelitis and septic arthritis -- Urinary tract infections -- Necrotizing enterocolitis and gastrointestinal infections -- Eye infections -- Skin and soft tissue infections -- Bacterial infections -- Mycoplasmas -- Fungal infections -- Viral infections -- Other congenital infections -- Breast milk -- Surveillance -- Infection control -- Developing countries -- Prevention of neonatal infections -- Neonatal antimicrobials. Subjects:

Communicable Diseases--Handbooks. Infant, Newborn, Diseases--therapy--Handbooks. Evidence-Based Medicine--Handbooks. Notes: Includes bibliographical references and index. Additional formats: Online version: Isaacs, David, 1950- author. Evidence-based neonatal infections Chichester, West Sussex, UK: John Wiley & Sons Inc., 2014 9781118636671 (DLC) 2013027365 Dewey class no.: 618.92/01 NLM class no.: WS 39 Other system no.: (DNLM)101611712 Content type: text Media type: unmediated Carrier type: volume

Evidence-based physical diagnosis LCCN: 2011040627 Type of material: Book Personal name: McGee, Steven R. Main title: Evidence-based physical diagnosis/Steven McGee. Edition: 3rd ed. Published/Created: Philadelphia: Elsevier/Saunders, c2012. Description: xv, 719 p.: ill.; 22 cm ISBN: 9781437722079 (pbk.: alk. paper) LC classification: RC76 .M347 2012 Subjects: Physical Examination--methods. Evidence-Based Medicine--methods. Notes: Includes bibliographical references and index. Dewey class no.: 616.07/54 NLM class no.: WB 200 Other system no.: (DNLM)101570116 Shelf Location: FLS2013 003255 CALL NUMBER: RC76 .M347 2012 OVERFLOWA5S Request in: Jefferson or Adams Building Reading Rooms (FLS1) CALL NUMBER: RC76 .M347 2012 LANDOVR Copy 2 Request in: Jefferson or Adams Building Reading Rooms - STORED OFFSITE

Evidence-based practice in audiology: evaluating interventions for children and adults with hearing impairment LCCN: 2011051391 Type of material: Book Main title: Evidence-based practice in audiology: evaluating interventions for children and adults with hearing impairment/Lena Wong and Louise Hickson. Published/Created: San Diego, CA: Plural Pub., c2012. Description: xiii, 339 p.: ill.; 26 cm. ISBN: 9781597564199 (alk. paper) 1597564192 (alk. paper) LC classification: RF290 .E77 2012 Related names: Wong, Lena. Hickson, Louise M. Contents: Evidence-based practice in audiology/Lena Wong and Louise Hickson -- Evaluating the evidence on audiologic interventions/Michael Valente, Maureen Valente, and

Laura Czarniak -- Matching evidence with client preferences/Ariane Laplante-Levesque, Louise Hickson, and Linda Worrall -- Hearing aids for adults/Larry E. Humes and Vidya Krull -- Hearing aids for children/Teresa Y.C. Ching -- Evidence-based practice and emerging new technologies/Gitte Keidser -- Evidence about the effectiveness of cochlear implants for adults/Richard Dowell -- Evidence about the effectiveness of cochlear implants for children: open-set speech recognition/Emily A. Tobey ... [et al.] -- Bimodal fitting or bilateral cochlear implantation?/Teresa Y.C. Ching and Paola Incerti -- Evidence about the effectiveness of aural rehabilitation programs for adults/Theresa Chisolm and Michelle Arnold -- Evidence about the effectiveness of treatments related to tinnitus/William Noble -- Evidence about the effectiveness of interventions for auditory processing disorder/Wayne J. Wilson and Wendy Arnott -- Evaluation and implementation of evidence-based practice in audiology/Lena Wong and Louise Hickson. Subjects: Hearing Disorders--therapy. Evidence-Based Medicine. Notes: Includes bibliographical references and index. Dewey class no.: 617.8 NLM class no.: WV 270 Other system no.: (DNLM)101574537 Shelf Location: FLM2013 000695 CALL NUMBER: RF290 .E77 2012 OVERFLOWA5S Request in: Jefferson or Adams Building Reading Rooms (FLM1)

Evidence-based practice of palliative medicine LCCN: 2012039834 Type of material: Book Main title: Evidence-based practice of palliative medicine/[edited by] Nathan E. Goldstein, R. Sean Morrison. Published/Created: Philadelphia: Elsevier/Saunders, c2013. Description: xxi, 499 p.: ill.; 28 cm. ISBN: 9781437737967 (pbk.: alk. paper) 143773796X (pbk.: alk. paper) LC classification: R726.8 .E928 2013 Related names: Goldstein, Nathan E. Morrison, R. Sean (Rolfe Sean) Subjects: Palliative treatment--Miscellanea. Evidence-based medicine--Miscellanea. Terminal care--Miscellanea. Palliative Care. Evidence-Based Medicine. Notes: Includes bibliographical references. Dewey class no.: 616.02/9 NLM class no.: WB 310 Other system no.: (DNLM)101593133 CALL NUMBER: R726.8 .E928 2013

Copy 1 Request in: Jefferson or Adams Building Reading Rooms

Evidence-based prevention LCCN: 2012040375 Type of material: Book Main title: Evidence-based prevention/Katherine Raczynski ... [et al.]. Published/Created: Thousand Oaks, Calif.: SAGE Publications, c2013. Description: viii, 83 p.; 26 cm. ISBN: 9781452258003 (pbk.) 1452258007 (pbk.) LC classification: RA790 .E935 2013 Related names: Raczynski, Katherine A. Subjects: Preventive mental health services. Evidence-based medicine. Notes: Includes bibliographical references (p. 75-79) and index. Series: Prevention practice kit Dewey class no.: 362.2/0425 Shelf Location: FLM2014 113238 CALL NUMBER: RA790 .E935 2013 OVERFLOWA5S Request in: Jefferson or Adams Building Reading Rooms (FLM1)

Evidence-based procedural dermatology LCCN: 2011938458 Type of material: Book Main title: Evidence-based procedural dermatology/Murad Alam, editor. Published/Created: New York: Springer, c2012. Description: xviii, 474 p.: ill. (chiefly col.); 26 cm. ISBN: 9780387094236 (hbk.: alk. paper) 0387094237 (hbk.: alk. paper) 9780387094243 (e-ISBN) 0387094245 (e-ISBN) LC classification: RL71 .E955 2012 Related names: Alam, Murad. Subjects: Skin--Diseases. Skin Diseases--therapy. Cosmetic Techniques. Evidence-Based Medicine. Reconstructive Surgical Procedures. Notes: Includes bibliographical references and index. Dewey class no.: 616.5 NLM class no.: 2012 B-820 WR 650 WR 650 E93 2012 National bib no.: GBB0C4677 National bib agency no.: 101579583 Other system no.: (OCoLC)ocn785706172 Shelf Location: FLM2013 016269 CALL NUMBER: RL71 .E955 2012 OVERFLOWA5S Request in: Jefferson or Adams Building Reading Rooms (FLM1)

Evidence-based public health practice LCCN: 2011039063 Type of material: Book Personal name: Fink, Arlene. Main title: Evidence-based public health practice/Arlene G. Fink. Published/Created: Thousand Oaks: Sage Publications, c2013. Description: xxiii, 298 p.: ill.; 23 cm. ISBN: 9781412997447 (pbk.) LC classification: RA440.85 .F56 2013 Subjects: Public health. Evidence-based medicine. Notes: Includes bibliographical references and index. Dewey class no.: 362.1 CALL NUMBER: RA440.85 .F56 2013 Copy 1 Request in: Jefferson or Adams Building Reading Rooms CALL NUMBER: RA440.85 .F56 2013 LANDOVR Copy 2 Request in: Jefferson or Adams Building Reading Rooms - STORED OFFSITE

Evidence-based rehabilitation: a guide to practice LCCN: 2013027660 Type of material: Book Main title: Evidence-based rehabilitation: a guide to practice/edited by Mary Law, PhD, OT Reg (Ont), FCAHS, School of Rehabilitation Science, McMaster University, Hamilton, Ontario, Canada, Joy C. MacDermid, PhD, PT Reg (Ont), FCAHS, School of Rehabilitation Science, McMaster University, Hamilton, Ontario, Canada. Edition: Third edition. Published/Produced: Thorofare, NJ, USA: Slack Incorporated, [2014] ©2014 Description: viii, 429 pages: illustrations; 27 cm ISBN: 9781617110214 (hbk.: alk. paper) LC classification: RM930 .E934 2014 Related names: Law, Mary C., editor of compilation. MacDermid, Joy, editor of compilation. Summary: "While evidence-based practice (EBP) has greatly influenced rehabilitation in the past decade, it continues to evolve and practitioners need guidance to implement evidence into their practice. Evidence-Based Rehabilitation: A Guide to Practice, the best-selling text providing step-by-step EBP guidance for rehabilitation professionals, has been updated into an expanded Third Edition. In Evidence-Based Rehabilitation, Third Edition Drs. Mary Law and Joy MacDermid, along with their contributors, explain evidence-based rehabilitation, the concepts underlying EBP, and build the reader's knowledge and skills through specific learning. The text is organized by the steps of the EBP process--introduction to EBP, finding the evidence, assessing the evidence, and using the evidence. EBP focuses first and foremost on making the best decisions for each client and using the best information available. For many rehabilitation practitioners, building skills in EBP is best done one step at a time. Evidence-Based Rehabilitation helps the rehabilitation student and practitioner develop his or her knowledge and skills to implement evidence-based rehabilitation in practice. Designed and written by an occupational therapist and a physical therapist with extensive research, education, and practice experience, Evidence-Based Rehabilitation: A Guide to Practice, Third Edition will guide both occupational therapy and physical therapy students and practitioners as they incorporate evidence-based practice into their work"--Provided by publisher. Contents: Introduction to evidence-based practice/Mary Law and Joy C. MacDermid -- Development of evidence-based knowledge/Winnie Dunn and Jill E. Foreman -- Becoming an evidence-based practitioner/Aliki Thomas and Annie McCluskey -- Outcome measurement in evidence-based rehabilitation/Joy C. MacDermid, Mary Law, and Susan L. Michlovitz -- Asking clinical questions and searching for the evidence/Jennie Q. Lou and Paola Durando -- Evaluating the evidence/Joy C. MacDermid and Mary Law -- Systematically reviewing the evidence/Laura Bradley and Mary Law -- Evaluating the evidence: economic evaluations/Mary Law, Michael Law, and Diane Watson -- Knowledge translation/Mary Law and Joy C. MacDermid -- Strategies to build evidence into practice/Mary Law and Joy C. MacDermid -- Evidence synthesis practice tools: guidelines, algorithms, clinical pathways, and decision aids/Joy C. MacDermid -- Communicating evidence to clients, managers, and funders/Linda Tickle-Degnen -- Moving evidence into practice: case examples of the knowledge-to-Action cycle at work/Jocelyn Harris, Saurabh Mehta, and Joy C. MacDermid. Subjects: Rehabilitation--methods. Evidence-Based Medicine--methods. Treatment Outcome. Notes: Includes bibliographical references and index. Dewey class no.: 617/.03 NLM class no.: WB 320 Other system no.: (DNLM)101612172 Content type: text Media type: unmediated Carrier type: volume Shelf Location: FLM2015 051205 CALL NUMBER: RM930 .E934 2014 OVERFLOWJ34 Request in: Jefferson or Adams Building Reading Rooms (FLM2)

Evidence-based research in pediatric nutrition LCCN: 2013025761 Type of material: Book Main title: Evidence-based research in pediatric nutrition/volume editors, Hania Szajewska,

Warsaw, Raanan Shamir, Petach-Tikva. Published/Produced: Basel; New York: Karger, 2013. Description: x, 111 pages: illustrations; 26 cm. ISBN: 9783318024562 (hard cover: alk. paper) LC classification: RJ53.P37 E95 2013 Related names: Szajewska, Hania, editor of compilation. Shamir, Raanan editor of compilation. Contents: Importance of systematic reviews and meta-analyses in pediatric nutrition/Szajewska, H. -- Strengths and weaknesses of observational nutritional trials/Patro-Go B., Szajewska, H. -- Scientific standards for human intervention trials evaluating health benefits of foods, and their application to infants, children, and adolescents/Woodside, J.V., Koletzko, B.V., Patterson, C.C., Welch, R.W. -- Early nutrition and health: short- and long-term outcomes/Gruszfeld, D., Socha, P. -- Probiotics, prebiotics, and dietary fiber in the management of functional gastrointestinal disorders/Horvath, A., Szajewska, H. -- Growing-up milk: a necessity or marketing?/Przyrembel, H, Agostoni, C. -- Cow's milk and goat's milk/Turck, T. -- The timing of introduction of complementary foods and later health/Agostoni, C., Przyrembel, H. -- Dietary interventions for primary allergy prevention - what is the evidence?/von Berg, A. -- Vitamin and mineral supplementation of term infants: are they necessary?/Lubetzky, R., Mandel, D., Mimouni, F.B. -- Enteral nutrition/Kolaek, S. -- Celiac disease - prevention strategies through early infant nutrition/Chmielewska, A., Szajewska, H., Shamir, R. -- Interventions for treating obesity in children/De Miguel-Etayo, P., Bueno, G., Garagorri, J.M., Moreno, L.A. Subjects: Child Nutritional Physiological Phenomena. Diet Therapy. Evidence-Based Medicine. Food. Notes: Includes bibliographical references and indexes. Series: World review of nutrition and dietetics, 0084-2230; vol. 108 World review of nutrition and dietetics; v. 108. 0084-2230 Dewey class no.: 615.8/548083 NLM class no.: W1 WO898 v.108 2013 WS 130 Other system no.: (DNLM)101611128 Invalid ISBN: 9783318024579 (electronic version) Content type: text Media type: unmediated Carrier type: volume Shelf Location: FLM2014 000611 CALL NUMBER: RJ53.P37 E95 2013 OVERFLOWA5S Request in:

Jefferson or Adams Building Reading Rooms (FLM1)

Evidence-guided practice: a framework for clinical decision making in athletic training LCCN: 2014046920 Type of material: Book Personal name: Van Lunen, Bonnie, author. Main title: Evidence-guided practice: a framework for clinical decision making in athletic training/Bonnie Van Lunen, Dorice A. Hankemeier, Cailee E. Welch. Published/Produced: Thorofare, NJ: Slack Incorporated, [2015] Projected pub date: 1502 Description: p.; cm. ISBN: 9781617116032 (paperback: alk. paper) LC classification: RC1211 Related names: Hankemeier, Dorice A., author. Welch, Cailee E., author. Summary: "Athletic trainers must have a foundation in the concepts of evidence-based practice to deliver patient care in an effective way. It is critical that students and clinicians formulate clinical plans that will be effective for individual patients. With that goal in mind, Evidence-Guided Practice: A Framework for Clinical Decision Making in Athletic Training teaches the athletic trainer that evidence-based practice concepts must be incorporated into daily clinical practice. Written in a conversational tone, Drs. Bonnie Van Lunen, Dorice Hankemeier, and Cailee Welch provide a practical and concise resource for athletic trainers to use when interpreting what the available evidence means for them and how it can be effectively applied in daily patient care. The competencies within athletic training and other health care professions were considered when each chapter was constructed. Special care was taken to include examples that are specific to athletic training and instructional applications for educators. The first of its kind, Evidence-Guided Practice: A Framework for Clinical Decision Making in Athletic Training is the only resource athletic training students, clinicians, or other health care professionals will need to properly put evidence-based concepts into practice"--Provided by publisher. Subjects: Sports Medicine--methods. Athletes. Athletic Performance. Evidence-Based Medicine. Notes: Includes bibliographical references and index. Dewey class no.: 617.1/027 NLM class no.: QT 261 Other system no.: (DNLM)101647556 Content type: text Media type: unmediated Carrier type: volume

Exploring immunology: concepts and evidence LCCN: 2014397005 Type of material: Book Personal name: MacPherson, Gordon (G. Gordon) Main title: Exploring immunology: concepts and evidence/Gordon MacPherson and Jon Austyn; illustrations by Ruth Hammelehle. Published/Created: Weinheim, Germany: Wiley-Blackwell, c2012. Description: xx, 357 p.: col. ill.; 29 cm. ISBN: 9783527324309 (hardcover: alk. paper) 3527324305 (hardcover: alk. paper) 9783527324125 (softcover: alk. paper) 3527324127 (softcover: alk. paper) Publisher no. 1132430 000 LC classification: QR181 .M323 2012 Related names: Austyn, Jonathan M. Contents: Immune system -- Infection and immunity -- Functional anatomy of the immune system -- Innate immunity -- T cell-mediated immunity -- Antibody-mediated immunity -- Immunity, disease and therapy. Subjects: Immunology. Evidence-based medicine. Notes: Includes index. NLM class no.: 2012 E-609 Other class no.: 610 National bib no.: GBB012699 09,N51,1382 National bib agency no.: 101586084 015479658 Other system no.: (OCoLC)ocn810115722 CALL NUMBER: QR181 .M323 2012 Copy 1 Request in: Jefferson or Adams Building Reading Rooms

Fundamentals of evidence-based medicine LCCN: 2013945419 Type of material: Book Main title: Fundamentals of evidence-based medicine/[edited by] Kameshwar Prasad. Published/Produced: New York: Springer, 2013. Projected pub date: 1308 Description: pages cm ISBN: 9788132208303 (hard cover: alk. paper) Content type: text Media type: unmediated Carrier type: volume

Fundamentals of geriatric pharmacotherapy LCCN: 2014034598 Type of material: Book Main title: Fundamentals of geriatric pharmacotherapy/[edited by] Lisa C. Hutchison, Rebecca B. Sleeper. Published/Produced: Bethesda, Maryland: American Society of Health-System Pharmacists, [2015] Projected pub date: 1503 Description: p.; cm. ISBN: 9781585284351 LC classification: RC953.7 Related names: Hutchison, Lisa C., editor. Sleeper, Rebecca B., editor. American Society of Health-System Pharmacists, issuing body. Contents: Challenges in geriatric care/Rebecca B. Sleeper --

Ethical and socioeconomic considerations/Susan W. Miller -- Biomedical principles of aging/Lisa C. Hutchison -- Geriatric assessment/Sunny A. Linnebur -- Adverse drug events, polypharmacy, and medication management/Joe T. Hanlon, Emily R. Hajjar, and Robert Maher -- Palliative and hospice care/Lindsey Dayer and Lisa C. Hutchison -- Cardiovascular disorders/Kristen M. Cook -- Respiratory disorders/Michael R. Brodeur -- Renal and urologic disorders/Erica L. Estus, Nicole J. Asal, and Norma J. Owens -- Endocrine disorders/Lisa Cohen, Anne L. Hume, and Christine Eisenhower -- Gastrointestinal disorders and nutrition/Lisa C. Hutchison, Rebecca B. Sleeper -- Central nervous system disorders/Amie Taggart Blaszczyk and Lisa C. Hutchison -- Psychiatric disorders/Monica Mathys and Myra T. Belgeri -- Pain and sensory disorders/Meri Hix -- Musculoskeletal and connective tissue disorders/Mary Beth O'Connell and Michelle Fritsch -- Anemia and preventive therapy/Sum Lam, Angela Cheng, and James Nawarskas -- Infections and antimicrobial stewardship/Rebecca B. Sleeper and Kelsey Van. Subjects: Drug Therapy. Geriatrics--methods. Aged. Evidence-Based Medicine--methods. Geriatric Assessment. Notes: Includes bibliographical references and index. Dewey class no.: 615.5/80846 NLM class no.: WT 166 Other system no.: (DNLM)101640218 Content type: text Media type: unmediated Carrier type: volume

Geriatric medicine: an evidence-based approach LCCN: 2014941934 Type of material: Book Main title: Geriatric medicine: an evidence-based approach/edited by Frank Lally, Christine Roffe. Edition: First edition. Published/Produced: New York, NY: Oxford University Press, 2014. Description: xiv, 221 pages: illustrations; 24 cm ISBN: 9780199689644 (pbk.) LC classification: RC952 .G3935 2014 Related names: Lally, Frank, editor. Roffe, Christine, editor. Subjects: Geriatrics. Older people--Medical care. Evidence-based medicine. Notes: Includes bibliographical references and index. Dewey class no.: 618.97 Content type: text Media type: unmediated Carrier type: volume CALL NUMBER: RC952 .G3935 2014 Copy 1 Request in: Reference -

Science Reading Room (Adams, 5th Floor)

Gestational diabetes: origins, complications, and treatment LCCN: 2013047331 Type of material: Book Uniform title: Gestational diabetes (Petry) Main title: Gestational diabetes: origins, complications, and treatment/editor, Clive J. Petry. Published/Produced: Boca Raton: Taylor & Francis /CRC Press, [2014] Description: vii, 227 pages: illustrations; 24 cm ISBN: 9781439879962 (hardcover: alk. paper) LC classification: RG580.D5 .G475 2014 Related names: Petry, Clive J., editor of compilation. Summary: "Discussing the origins, care, and consequences of gestational diabetes mellitus (GDM), this book focuses on evidence-based medicine to highlight various aspects of this rapidly growing condition. It provides glucose requirements for fetal growth and maternal and fetal metabolism as well as insulin secretion and sensitivity in pregnancy; covers genetic risk factors, autoimmunity, interaction with obesity, and associations with fetal growth genes; presents diet therapies and the role of exercise and nutrition; and reviews the effects of rapid-, short-, and long-acting insulin, oral hypoglycemic agents in pregnancy, and clinical approaches"--Provided by publisher. Subjects: Diabetes, Gestational. Evidence-Based Medicine. Notes: Includes bibliographical references and index. Dewey class no.: 618.3/646 NLM class no.: WQ 248 Other system no.: (DNLM)101620998 Content type: text Media type: unmediated Carrier type: volume Shelf Location: FLM2014 167191 CALL NUMBER: RG580.D5 .G475 2014 OVERFLOWA5S Request in: Jefferson or Adams Building Reading Rooms (FLM1)

Health care operations and supply chain management: operations, planning, and control LCCN: 2012033935 Type of material: Book Personal name: Kros, John F. Main title: Health care operations and supply chain management: operations, planning, and control/John F. Kros, Evelyn C. Brown. Edition: First edition. Published/Produced: San Francisco: Jossey-Bass, a Wiley imprint, [2013] Description: xxxii, 542 pages: illustrations; 24 cm ISBN: 9781118109779 (pbk.) LC classification: RA971.3 .K767 2013 Related names: Brown, Evelyn C., 1966-

Summary: "This resource provides students with a thorough foundation in operations management, supply chain management, and the strategic implementation of programs, techniques, and tools for reducing costs and improving quality in health care organizations. It incorporates the features and functions of Microsoft Excel where appropriate in its coverage of supply chain strategy, process design and analysis of health care operations, managing health care operations quality, and planning and controlling health care operations. The book illustrates leading edge concepts and techniques such as six-sigma and lean logistics, and shows how operations and process improvement relate to contemporary health care trends such as evidence-based medicine and pay-for-performance"--Provided by publisher. Subjects: Health facilities--Business management. Health services administration. MEDICAL/Administration. Notes: Includes bibliographical references and index. Dewey class no.: 362.1068 Other class no.: MED002000 Content type: text Media type: unmediated Carrier type: volume Shelf Location: FLM2013 000819 CALL NUMBER: RA971.3 .K767 2013 OVERFLOWA5S Request in: Jefferson or Adams Building Reading Rooms (FLM1) CALL NUMBER: RA971.3 .K767 2013 LANDOVR Copy 2 Request in: Jefferson or Adams Building Reading Rooms - STORED OFFSITE

Hospital-based palliative medicine: a practical, evidence-based approach LCCN: 2014034458 Type of material: Book Main title: Hospital-based palliative medicine: a practical, evidence-based approach/edited by Steven Pantilat, Wendy Anderson, Matthew Gonzales, Eric Widera. Published/Produced: Hoboken, New Jersey: John Wiley & Sons Inc., 2015. Projected pub date: 1503 Description: p.; cm. ISBN: 9781118772577 (paperback) LC classification: R726.8 Related names: Pantilat, Steven, editor. Anderson, Wendy, editor. Gonzales, Matthew, editor. Widera, Eric, editor. Summary: "Hospital-Based Palliative Medicine: A Practical, Evidence-Based Approach focuses on improving a Hospitalist's ability to provide quality palliative care in the inpatient hospital setting. Although several large textbooks exist for the palliative care provider, there are few detailed resources aimed specifically at the general Hospitalist and hospital-based staff. Existing textbooks dedicate at most only one chapter to palliative care and they lack the detail and specificity in symptom management and communication skills to truly guide care. Hospital-Based Palliative Medicine addresses each of the major components involved in the delivery of inpatient palliative care. These include the management of complex symptoms and the use of specific communication techniques - right down to the actual words to say to the patient - to convey important information such as the reason for and use of medication and how to handle difficult topics with patients and their families and caregivers. The book's authors are all leaders in the field of palliative care, and most of them also practice as hospitalists, and thus understand both perspectives. Chapters are presented in a consistent format with particular attention to both clinical pearls and pitfalls, making the material practical and easily accessible to the busy hospitalist and associated hospital staff"--Provided by publisher. Subjects: Palliative Care--methods. Evidence-Based Medicine--methods. Hospitals. Notes: Includes bibliographical references and index. Additional formats: Online version: Hospital-based palliative medicine Hoboken, New Jersey: John Wiley & Sons Inc., 2015 9781118772584 (DLC) 2014034944 Series: Hospital medicine, current concepts; 8 Hospital medicine, current concepts; 8. Dewey class no.: 616.02/9 NLM class no.: WB 310 Other system no.: (DNLM)101640170 Content type: text Media type: unmediated Carrier type: volume

How to read a paper: the basics of evidence-based medicine LCCN: 2013038474 Type of material: Book Personal name: Greenhalgh, Trisha, author. Main title: How to read a paper: the basics of evidence-based medicine/Trisha Greenhalgh. Edition: Fifth edition. Published/Produced: Chichester, West Sussex: John Wiley & Sons Inc., 2014. Projected pub date: 1405 Description: p.; cm. ISBN: 9781118800966 (pbk.) LC classification: R118.6 Contents: Why read papers at all? -- Searching the literature -- Getting your bearings: what is this paper about? -- Assessing methodological quality --

Statistics for the non-statistician -- Papers that report trials of drugs and other simple interventions -- Papers that report trials of complex interventions -- Papers that report diagnostic or screening tests -- Papers that summarise other papers (systematic reviews and meta-analyses) -- Papers that tell you what to do (guidelines) -- Papers that tell you what things cost (economic analyses) -- Papers that go beyond numbers (qualitative research) -- Papers that report questionnaire research -- Papers that report quality improvement case studies -- Getting evidence into practice. Subjects: Evidence-Based Practice. Journalism, Medical. Research. Notes: Includes bibliographical references and index. Additional formats: Online version: Greenhalgh, Trisha, author. How to read a paper Fifth edition. Chichester, West Sussex: John Wiley & Sons Inc., 2014 9781118801093 (DLC) 2013039190 Dewey class no.: 610.72 NLM class no.: WB 102.5 Other system no.: (DNLM)101617639 Content type: text Media type: unmediated Carrier type: volume

Identifying perinatal depression and anxiety: evidence-based practice in screening, psychosocial assessment and management LCCN: 2014048416 Type of material: Book Main title: Identifying perinatal depression and anxiety: evidence-based practice in screening, psychosocial assessment and management/edited by Jeannette Milgrom, Alan Gemmill. Published/Produced: Chichester, UK; Malden, MA: John Wiley & Sons Inc., 2015. Projected pub date: 1507 Description: p.; cm. ISBN: 9781118509654 (hb) 9781118509692 (pb) LC classification: RC537 Related names: Milgrom, Jeannette, editor. Gemmill, Alan, editor. Summary: "Identifying Perinatal Depression and Anxiety brings together the very latest research and clinical practice on this topic from around the world in one valuable resource. Examines current screening and management models, particularly those in Australia, England and Wales, Scotland, and the United States. Discusses the evidence, accuracy, and limitations of screening methods in the context of challenges, policy issues, and questions that require further research. Up to date practical guidance of how to screen, assess, diagnose and manage is provided. Considers the importance of screening processes that involve infants and fathers, additional training for health professionals, pathways to care following screening, and the economics of screening. Offers forward-thinking synthesis and analysis of the current state of the field by leading international experts, with the goal of sketching out areas in need of future research"--Provided by publisher. Subjects: Depression, Postpartum--diagnosis. Anxiety Disorders--diagnosis. Anxiety Disorders--psychology. Depression, Postpartum--psychology. Evidence-Based Medicine--methods. Internationality. Notes: Includes bibliographical references and index. Additional formats: Online version: Identifying perinatal depression and anxiety Chichester, UK; Malden, MA: John Wiley & Sons Inc., 2015 9781118509685 (DLC) 2014050001 Dewey class no.: 616.85/27 NLM class no.: WQ 500 Other system no.: (DNLM)101648275 Content type: text Media type: unmediated Carrier type: volume

Inflammatory bowel disease: an evidence-based practical guide LCCN: 2012360778 Type of material: Book Main title: Inflammatory bowel disease: an evidence-based practical guide/edited by Ailsa L. Hart, Siew C. Ng. Edition: 1st ed. Published/Created: Harley, UK: TFM, c2012. Description: x, 292 p.: ill.; 21 cm. ISBN: 9781903378823 1903378826 LC classification: RC862.I53 I52326 2012 Related names: Hart, Ailsa L. Ng, Siew Chin. Subjects: Inflammatory bowel diseases--Treatment. Inflammatory bowel diseases--Treatment--Complications. Inflammatory Bowel Diseases--therapy. Evidence-Based Medicine--methods. Notes: Includes bibliographical references. Dewey class no.: 616.3/44 NLM class no.: 2012 C-187 WI 420 WI 420 I43 2012 National bib no.: GBB115717 National bib agency no.: 101580556 015744226 Other system no.: (OCoLC)ocn778323643 Shelf Location: FLS2013 020430 CALL NUMBER: RC862.I53 I52326 2012 OVERFLOWA5S Request in: Jefferson or Adams Building Reading Rooms (FLS1)

Interprofessional rehabilitation: a person-centred approach LCCN: 2012015864 Type of material: Book Main title: Interprofessional rehabilitation: a person-centred approach/edited by Sarah G. Dean, Richard J. Siegert, William J. Taylor. Published/Created: Chichester, West Sussex; Ames, Iowa: Wiley-Blackwell, 2012. Description: xviii, 195 p.: ill.; 25 cm. ISBN: 9780470655962 (pbk.: alk. paper) LC classification: RM930 .I58 2012 Related names: Dean, Sarah G. Siegert, Richard J. Taylor, William J., 1964- Contents: Introduction: interprofessional rehabilitation - a person-centred approach/Richard J. Siegert, William Taylor, and Sarah G. Dean -- A rehabilitation framework: the international classification of functioning, disability and health/William J. Taylor and Szilvia Geyh -- An interprofessional approach to rehabilitation/Sarah G. Dean and Claire Ballinger -- Processes in rehabilitation/William Levack and Sarah G. Dean -- Outcome measurement in rehabilitation/Richard J. Siegert and Jo Adams -- The person in context/Julie Pryor and Sarah G. Dean -- Conclusion: interprofessional rehabilitation a person-centred approach/Sarah G. Dean, Richard J. Siegert, and William J. Taylor. Subjects: Rehabilitation--psychology. Evidence-Based Medicine. Patient Care Team. Treatment Outcome. Notes: Includes bibliographical references and index. Dewey class no.: 616.86/03 NLM class no.: WB 320 Other system no.: (DNLM)101582555 Shelf Location: FLM2013 001805 CALL NUMBER: RM930 .I58 2012 OVERFLOWA5S Request in: Jefferson or Adams Building Reading Rooms (FLM1)

Intra-uterine insemination: evidence-based guidelines for daily practice LCCN: 2013036751 Type of material: Book Main title: Intra-uterine insemination: evidence-based guidelines for daily practice/edited by Ben Cohlen, MD, PhD, Fertility Center Isala, Zwolle, The Netherlands, Willem Ombelet, MD, PhD, Institute for Fertility Technology, Ziekenhuis Oost Limburg, Genk, Belgium. Published/Produced: Boca Raton: CRC Press/Taylor & Francis Group, [2014] Description: xiii, 206 pages: illustrations; 26 cm. ISBN: 9781841849881 (pbk.: acid-free paper) LC classification: RG134 .I58 2014 Related names: Cohlen, Ben, 1963- editor of compilation. Ombelet, W. (Willem), editor of compilation. Summary: "Intra-uterine insemination (IUI) is a widely used fertility treatment for couples with unexplained and male subfertility. Although it is less invasive and less expensive as athan several other treatment options, than in vitro fertilization, severalsome points about the factors affecting its outcome IUI remain controversial and there remains concern about some of the possible aspects of treatmentside-effects, such as an increase in multiple pregnancy rates. This is a comprehensive evidence-based book from an international IUI expert team, with guidelines for daily practice clearly stated and summarized for readers convenience"--Provided by publisher. Subjects: Insemination, Artificial--methods. Evidence-Based Medicine--standards. Infertility--therapy. Treatment Outcome. Notes: Includes bibliographical references and index. Series: Reproductive medicine and assisted reproductive techniques Reproductive medicine & assisted reproductive techniques series. Dewey class no.: 618.1/78 NLM class no.: WQ 208 Other system no.: (DNLM)101616847 Content type: text Media type: unmediated Carrier type: volume Shelf Location: FLM2014 020353 CALL NUMBER: RG134 .I58 2014 OVERFLOWA5S Request in: Jefferson or Adams Building Reading Rooms (FLM1)

Introduction to nursing research: incorporating evidence-based practice LCCN: 2012035427 Type of material: Book Personal name: Boswell, Carol. Main title: Introduction to nursing research: incorporating evidence-based practice/edited by Carol Boswell, Sharon Cannon. Edition: 3rd ed. Published/Created: Burlington, MA: Jones & Bartlett Learning, c2014. Description: xviii, 489 p.: ill.; 23 cm. ISBN: 9781449681968 (pbk.) 9781449695071 LC classification: RT81.5 .B68 2014 Related names: Boswell, Carol. Cannon, Sharon, 1940- Contents: Connection between research and evidence-based practice -- Overview of evidence -- Overview of research -- Ethics for nursing research and evidence-based practice -- Picot, problem statement, research question, hypothesis -- Literature review: searching and writing the evidence -- Sampling -- Quantitative research design -- Qualitative and mixed research methods -- Data collection -- Reliability, validity, and trustworthiness -- Data analysis -- The research critique process and the evidence-based appraisal process -- Translational research and practical applications -- Application of evidence-based nursing practice with research. Subjects: Nursing Research--methods. Evidence-Based Medicine. Notes: Includes bibliographical references and index. Includes bibliographical references and index. Dewey class no.: 610.72 Other system no.: (DNLM)101591299 Shelf Location: FLM2014 002918 CALL NUMBER: RT81.5 .B68 2014 OVERFLOWA5S Request in: Jefferson or Adams Building Reading Rooms (FLM1)

Knowledge translation in health care: moving from evidence to practice LCCN: 2013011462 Type of material: Book Main title: Knowledge translation in health care: moving from evidence to practice/edited by Sharon E. Straus, Jacqueline Tetroe, Ian D. Graham. Edition: 2nd ed. Published/Created: Chichester, West Sussex; Hoboken, NJ: Wiley/BMJ Books, 2013. Description: xvii, 406 p.: illustrations; 22 cm. ISBN: 9781118413548 (pbk.) LC classification: R723.7 .K663 2013 Related names: Straus, Sharon E. Tetroe, Jacqueline. Graham, Ian D. Subjects: Evidence-Based Medicine. Diffusion of Innovation. Information Dissemination. Notes: Includes bibliographical references and index. Additional formats: Online version: Knowledge translation in health care 2nd ed. Chichester, West Sussex: John Wiley & Sons, 2013 9781118413562 (DLC) 2013012012 Dewey class no.: 610 NLM class no.: WB 102.5 Other system no.: (DNLM)101604476 Shelf Location: FLS2014 023448 CALL NUMBER: R723.7 .K663 2013 OVERFLOWA5S Request in: Jefferson or Adams Building Reading Rooms (FLS1)

Lecture notes. Epidemiology, evidence-based medicine, and public health LCCN: 2012025764 Type of material: Book Personal name: Ben-Shlomo, Yoav. Main title: Lecture notes. Epidemiology, evidence-based medicine, and public health/Yoav Ben-Shlomo, Sara Brookes, Matthew Hickman. Edition: 6th ed. Published/Created: Chichester, West Sussex: John Wiley & Sons, 2013. Description: ix, 238 p.: col. ill.; 24 cm. ISBN: 9781444334784 (pbk.: alk. paper) LC classification: RA651 .B467 2013 Variant title: Epidemiology, evidence-based medicine, and public health Related names: Brookes, Sara. Hickman, Matthew. Farmer, R. D. T. Lecture notes. Epidemiology and public health medicine. Contents: Epidemiology: defining disease and normality/Sara Brookes & Yoav Ben-Shlomo -- Measuring and summarising data/Sara Brookes & Yoav Ben-Shlomo -- Epidemiological concepts/Sara Brookes & Yoav Ben-Shlomo -- Statistical inference, confidence intervals, and P values/Kate Tilling, Sara Brookes & Jonathan A.C. Sterne -- Observational studies/Mona Jeffreys & Yoav Ben-Shlomo -- Genetic epidemiology/David M. Evans & Ian Day -- Investigating causes of disease/Debbie A. Lawlor & John Macleod -- Evidence based medicine: an overview/Yoav Ben-Shlomo & Matthew Hickman -- Diagnosis/Penny Whiting & Richard M. Martin -- Prognosis/Yoav Ben-Shlomo & Matthew Hickman -- Effectiveness/Sara Brookes & Jenny Donovan -- Systematic reviews and meta-analysis/Penny Whiting & Jonathan A.C. Sterne -- Health economics/William Hollingworth & Sian Noble -- Audit, research ethics, and governance/Joanne Simon & Yoav Ben-Shlomo -- Public health/Matthew Hickman, Ruth Kipping & David Gunnell -- Screening/Angela E. Raffle -- Infectious disease epidemiology and surveillance/Caroline Trotter, Isabel Oliver & Matthew Hickman -- Inequalities in health/Bruna Galobardes, Mona Jeffreys & George Davey Smith -- Health improvement/Bruce Bolam -- Evaluating public health and complex interventions/Yoav Ben-Shlomo & Rona Campbell -- Health care targets/Maya Gobin & Gabriel Scally -- Global health/Sanjay Kinra, David L. Heymann & Shah Ebrahim. Subjects: Epidemiology. Epidemiologic Methods. Evidence-Based Medicine. Public Health. Notes: Rev. ed. of: Lecture notes. Epidemiology and public health medicine/Richard Farmer, Ross Lawrenson. 5th. 2004. Includes bibliographical references and index. Dewey class no.: 614.4 NLM class no.: WA 950 Other system no.: (DNLM)101586862 Shelf Location: FLM2013 031394 CALL NUMBER: RA651 .B467 2013 OVERFLOWA5S Request in: Jefferson or Adams Building Reading Rooms (FLM1)

Life cycle nutrition: an evidence-based approach LCCN: 2013038802 Type of material: Book Main title: Life cycle nutrition: an evidence-based approach/Sari Edelstein, PhD, RD, Department of Nutrition, Simmons College, Boston, Massachusetts. Edition: Second edition. Published/Produced: Burlington, Massachusetts: Jones & Bartlett Learning, [2015] ©2015 Description: xxxii, 559 pages; 28 cm ISBN: 9781449694302 (pbk.: alk. paper) 1449694306 (pbk.: alk. paper) 9781284036671 (pbk.: with access code) 1284036677 (pbk.: with access code) LC classification: QP141 .L53 2015 Related names: Edelstein, Sari, editor of compilation. Contents: Nutrition requirements during pregnancy -- Evidence-based nutrition in the life cycle: prenatal to the adolescent -- Normal infant nutrition -- Normal nutrition for toddler through school-aged children and the role of parents in promoting healthy nutrition in early childhood -- Normal adolescent nutrition -- Special topics in prenatal and infant nutrition: genetics and inborn errors of metabolism and failure to thrive -- Special topics in toddler and preschool nutrition: vitamins and minerals in childhood and children with disabilities -- Special topics in school-aged nutrition: pediatric vegetarianism, childhood obesity, and food allergies -- Special topics in preadolescence and adolescent nutrition: dietary guidelines for athletes, pediatric diabetes, and disordered eating -- Adult evidence-based nutrition in the life cycle -- Special topics in adult nutrition: chronic disease nutritional assessment -- Special topics in adults and chronic diseases: nutrition and public health -- Special topics in adult nutrition: physical activity and weight management -- Special topics in nutrition and the older adult: diet, life-style, disease, and pharmacologic considerations -- Special topics in age-related risks: unique nutrition issues in the older adult -- Special topics related to the registered dietitian and older adults: roles and responsibilities of the registered dietitian in long-term care -- Special topics in nutrition and ethics: feeding and ethical issues at the end of life -- Online -- Interpreting evidence-based research: major pediatric and adult nutrition studies. Subjects: Nutritional Physiological Phenomena. Evidence-Based Medicine. Human Development--physiology. Longitudinal

Studies. Notes: Includes bibliographical references and index. Dewey class no.: 612.3/9 NLM class no.: QU 145 Other system no.: (DNLM)101617756 Content type: text Media type: unmediated Carrier type: volume Shelf Location: FLM2014 127829 CALL NUMBER: QP141 .L53 2015 OVERFLOWA5S Request in: Jefferson or Adams Building Reading Rooms (FLM1)

Managing hot flushes with group cognitive behaviour therapy: an evidence based treatment manual for health professionals LCCN: 2014024381 Type of material: Book Personal name: Hunter, Myra, author. Main title: Managing hot flushes with group cognitive behaviour therapy: an evidence based treatment manual for health professionals/Myra Hunter and Melanie Smith. Published/Produced: Hove, East Sussex; New York, NY: Routledge, 2015. Projected pub date: 1111 Description: p.; cm. ISBN: 9781138026148 (hbk) 9781138026155 (pbk) LC classification: RC489.C62 Related names: Smith, Melanie, 1975-, author. Contents: Psychoeducation and the cognitive behavioural model -- Stress management, improving wellbeing and identifying precipitants -- Managing hot flushes using a cognitive behavioural approach -- Managing night sweats and improving sleep (part one) -- Managing night sweats and sleep (part two) -- Review and maintaining changes. Subjects: Cognitive Therapy--methods. Hot Flashes--therapy. Evidence-Based Medicine. Psychotherapy, Group--methods. Notes: Includes bibliographical references and index. Dewey class no.: 616.89/1425 NLM class no.: WP 580 Other system no.: (DNLM)101637341 Invalid ISBN: 9781315764191 (ebk) Content type: text Media type: unmediated Carrier type: volume CALL NUMBER: RC489.C62 Request in: Jefferson or Adams Building Reading Rooms

Maternal-fetal evidence-based guidelines LCCN: 2011025732 Type of material: Book Main title: Maternal-fetal evidence-based guidelines/edited by Vincenzo Berghella. Edition: 2nd ed. Published/Created: New York: Informa Healthcare, c2012. Projected pub date: 1110 Description: p.; cm. ISBN: 9781841848228 (hardback: alk. paper) LC classification: RG101 .M36 2012 Related names: Berghella, Vincenzo. Summary:

"Maternal-Fetal Medicine Evidence-Based Guidelines reviews the evidence for best practice in maternal-fetal medicine. It presents the reader with the right information, in the right format, by summarizing evidence in easy-to-use tables and algorithms. Each guideline is designed to "make it easy to do it right", with appropriate use of proven interventions and no use of harmful interventions. Plenty of evidence is available so that well-informed clinicians can reduce errors, so that the first aim is ultimately to improve the health of mother and fetus by providing quality care"-- Provided by publisher. Subjects: Obstetrics. Evidence-based medicine. Pregnancy Complications. Evidence-Based Medicine. Fetal Diseases. Notes: Includes bibliographical references and index. Series: Series in maternal fetal medicine Series in maternal-fetal medicine. Dewey class no.: 618.2 NLM class no.: WQ 240 Other system no.: (DNLM)101562779

Medical illuminations: using evidence, visualization and statistical thinking to improve healthcare LCCN: 2013938497 Type of material: Book Personal name: Wainer, Howard, author. Main title: Medical illuminations: using evidence, visualization and statistical thinking to improve healthcare/Howard Wainer, National Board of Medical Examiners. Edition: First edition. Published/Produced: Oxford, United Kingdom; New York, NY, United States of America: Oxford University Press, 2014. Description: xv, 175 pages: illustrations (some colour), maps (some colour); 24 cm ISBN: 9780199668793 (hbk.) 0199668795 (hbk.) LC classification: RA407 .W35 2014 Contents: New York's cancer maps: what we don't know won't hurt us, it's what we do know that ain't -- A centenary celebration for Will Burtin: a pioneer of scientific visualization -- That's funny ... -- Commentary on some graphs in the 2008 National Healthcare Quality Report -- Improving graphic displays by controlling creativity -- Diabetes and the obesity: taking a better look at blood sugar as a start -- A second look at second opinions, with hip fractures as an example -- False positives or is a pound of prevention worth an ounce of cure -- Assessing long-term risk with shorter-term data -- A remarkable horse: an inquiry into the accuracy of medical predictions -- On the role of replication in the advance of science: the survival of the fittist -- What does it take to change practice? -- Why is a raven like a writing desk? Musing on the power of convention. Subjects: Medical statistics. Evidence-based medicine. Statistics--Graphic methods. Notes: Includes bibliographical references (pages 155-170) and index. Dewey class no.: 610.21 National bib no.: GBB370955 National bib agency no.: 016471940 Other system no.: (OCoLC)ocn861313615 Content type: text Media type: unmediated Carrier type: volume Shelf Location: FLM2014 023576 CALL NUMBER: RA407 .W35 2014 OVERFLOWA5S Request in: Jefferson or Adams Building Reading Rooms (FLM1)

Medical research essentials LCCN: 2013043238 Type of material: Book Personal name: Esteitie, Rania, author. Main title: Medical research essentials/Rania Esteitie. Published/Produced: New York: McGraw-Hill Education Medical, [2014] Description: xi, 104 pages: illustrations; 24 cm ISBN: 9780071781640 (pbk.: alk. paper) 0071781641 (pbk.: alk. paper) LC classification: R850 .E88 2014 Contents: How to classify research studies -- Journal club -- How to interpret research -- How to plan research -- How to organize research -- How to present your research -- Deciphering different research domains. Subjects: Biomedical Research. Evidence-Based Medicine. Research Design. Notes: Includes bibliographical references and index. Dewey class no.: 610.72/4 NLM class no.: WB 25 Other system no.: (DNLM)101618994 Content type: text Media type: unmediated Carrier type: volume Shelf Location: FLM2014 165951 CALL NUMBER: R850 .E88 2014 OVERFLOWA5S Request in: Jefferson or Adams Building Reading Rooms (FLM1)

Mistletoe: from mythology to evidence-based medicine LCCN: 2015008686 Type of material: Book Uniform title: Mistletoe (Zänker) Main title: Mistletoe: from mythology to evidence-based medicine/volume editors, Kurt S. Zänker, Srini V. Kaveri. Published/Produced: Basel; New York: Karger, 2015. Projected pub date: 1506 Description: p.; cm. ISBN: 9783318054446 (hard cover: alk. paper) LC classification: RS431.A64

Related names: Zänker, Kurt S., editor. Kaveri, Srini V., editor. Contents: Mistletoe through cultural and medical history: the all-healing plant proves to be a cancer-specific remedy/Ramm, H. -- Chemical constituents of viscum album L.: implications for the pharmaceutical preparation of mistletoe/Urech, K.; Baumgartner, S. -- The anti-cancer activity of mistletoe preparations, as related to their polyphenolic profiles/Schramm, H.M. -- From Berlin and Witten to Southampton and Hamburg: 25 years of mistletoe research cooperation/Schumacher, U.; Pfüller, U. -- Mistletoe compounds as anti-cancer drugs: effects and mechanisms in the treatment of glioblastoma/Schötterl, S.; Naumann, U. -- Cancer surgery and supportive mistletoe therapy: from scepticism to randomised clinical trials/Galun, D.; Tröger, W.; Milicevic, M. -- Dissecting the anti-inflammatory effects of viscum album: inhibition of cytokine-induced expression of cyclo-oxygenase-2 and secretion of prostaglandin E2/Elluru, S.R.; Saha, C.; Hedge, P.; Friboulet, A.; Bayry, J.; Kaveri, S.V. -- Dancing with the Devil: cancer-related fatigue, from inflammation to treatment options/Zänker, K.S. Subjects: Antineoplastic Agents, Phytogenic--therapeutic use. Viscum album. Anti-Inflammatory Agents--therapeutic use. Fatigue--drug therapy. Notes: Includes bibliographical references and indexes. Series: Translational research in biomedicine, 1662-405X; v. 4 Translational research in biomedicine; v. 4. 1662-405X Dewey class no.: 615.7/98 NLM class no.: QZ 267 Other system no.: (DNLM)101653156 Invalid ISBN: 9783318054453 (e-ISBN) Content type: text Media type: unmediated Carrier type: volume

Neurogenic disorders of language and cognition: evidence-based clinical practice LCCN: 2013035668 Type of material: Book Personal name: Murray, Laura L., author. Uniform title: Neurogenic disorders of language Main title: Neurogenic disorders of language and cognition: evidence-based clinical practice/by Laura L. Murray, Heather M. Clark. Edition: Second edition. Published/Produced: Austin, Texas: Pro-Ed, an international publisher, [2015] ©2015 Description: xv, 641 pages: illustrations; 25 cm. + 1 DVD-ROM (4 3/4 in.) ISBN:

9781416405856 (pbk.) 1416405852 (pbk.) LC classification: RC423 .M753 2015 Related names: Clark, Heather M., author. Contents: Introduction: models and concepts -- Overview of neurogenic language and cognitive disorders -- Neuropathology of neurogenic language and cognitive disorders -- A general model of assessment -- Identifying complicating conditions -- Assessment of body structure and function: quantifying and qualifying linguistic disorders -- Assessment of body structure and function: quantifying and qualifying cognitive disorders -- Assessment of activity, participation, and quality of life -- Remediation of body structure and function: behavioral approaches for linguistic disorders -- Remediation of body structure and function: behavioral approaches for cognitive disorders -- Remediation of body structure and function: pharmacotherapy approaches -- Remediation of activity and participation: approaches for linguistic and cognitive disorders -- The context of care: legislative and economic influences. Subjects: Language Disorders--diagnosis. Language Disorders--therapy. Brain Diseases--complications. Cognition Disorders--diagnosis. Cognition Disorders--therapy. Evidence-Based Medicine--methods. Notes: Preceded by Neurogenic disorders of language: theory driven clinical practice/Laura L. Murray, Heather M. Clark. 2006. Includes bibliographical references. Dewey class no.: 616.85/5 NLM class no.: WL 340.2 Other system no.: (DNLM)101616259 Content type: text Media type: unmediated Carrier type: volume CALL NUMBER: RC423 .M753 2015 Copy 1 Request in: See Reference Staff. By Appt in Jefferson Main RR (MRC)

Neuroimaging and psychosocial addiction treatment: an integrative guide for researchers and clinicians LCCN: 2015002973 Type of material: Book Main title: Neuroimaging and psychosocial addiction treatment: an integrative guide for researchers and clinicians/edited by Sarah W. Feldstein Ewing, Assistant Professor, University of New Mexico, USA, Katie Witkiewitz, Associate Professor, University of New Mexico, USA, and Francesca M. Filbey, Associate Professor, University of Texas, USA . Published/Produced: New

York: Palgrave Macmillan, 2015. Projected pub date: 1505 Description: pages cm Links: Google. https://www.google.com/#q=%22Smoking%2C+Addiction+and+the+Offspring+Brain%22 ISBN: 9781137362643 (hardback) LC classification: RC564 .N475 2015 Related names: Feldstein Ewing, Sarah W., 1976- editor. Witkiewitz, Katie, editor. Filbey, Francesca M., 1972- editor. Summary: "Addiction might be an age-old affliction but we still only have a modest understanding of how and why addiction treatment works. This book uses an innovative translational approach to weave together basic biological (brain) mechanisms with human behaviour in order to provide a critical insight into why people do (and do not) change in the context of addiction treatment. With sections focusing on both adults and adolescents, this book bridges the gap between experimental scientists and clinical practitioners to provide an overview of the influence of basic brain functions. "-- Provided by publisher. Contents: Machine generated contents note: -- Preface -- PART I: INTRODUCTION -- 1. Translational Approaches to Addiction Treatment; Sarah W. Yip, Kathleen M. Carroll and Marc N. Potenza -- 2. Fundamentals of Addiction Neuroscience; Ariel Ketcherside and Francesca M. Filbey -- PART II: TRANSLATIONAL APPROACHES WITH ADULTS -- 3. Using Clinical Neuroscience to Understand Addiction Treatment; Joseph P. Schacht and Kent E. Hutchison -- 4. Neuropsychopharmacology in Addiction Treatment; Lara A. Ray, Kelly E. Courtney, Daniel Roche, and Karen Miotto -- 5. The Promise of Repetitive Transcranial Magnetic Stimulation to Treat Addiction; Rachel A. Rabin, Daniel M. Blumberger, Zafiris J. Daskalakis, Tony P. George, and Mera S. Barr -- 6. Neuroscience and Mindfulness-Based Interventions: Translating Neural Mechanisms to Addiction Treatment; Matthew R. Pearson, Corey R. Roos, David B. Brown, and Katie Witkiewitz -- 7. New Approaches to Treating Cannabis Dependence: From Neuroscience to Practice; Janna Cousijn and Francesca M. Filbey -- 8. Morphometric Biomarkers of Addiction and Treatment Response; Teresa R. Franklin, Joel Mumma, Kanchana Jagannathan, Reagan R. Wetherill, and Anna Rose

Childress -- 9. Neural Mechanisms Supporting the Regulation of Cigarette Craving; Stephen J. Wilson -- 10. Neuroeconomics: Implications for Understanding and Treating Addictive Behavior; David P. Jarmolowicz, Derek D. Reed, and Warren K. Bickel -- 11. Using Neuroimaging to Improve Emotion Regulation Treatments for Substance Use Disorders; Claire E. Wilcox and Bryon Adinoff -- PART III: TRANSLATIONAL APPROACHES WITH ADOLESCENTS -- 12. Introduction to Functional Brain Connectivity: Potential Contributions to Understanding Adolescent Vulnerability to Substance Abuse; Monique Ernst, Elizabeth A. Hale, Nicholas Balderston, Salvatore Torrisi -- 13. Approaching Adolescent Substance Abuse Treatment through Neuroscience; Anita Cservenka, Tam T. Nguyen-Louie, Susan F. Tapert, and Bonnie J. Nagel -- 14. Prenatal Exposure to Maternal Cigarette Smoking, Addiction and the Offspring Brain; Tomáš Paus and Zdenka Pausova -- 15. Deconstructing the Neural Substrates of Motivational Interviewing: A New Look at Unresolved Questions; Sarah W. Feldstein Ewing, Hollis Karoly, and Jon M. Houck -- 16. Neural Influences in Contingency Management for Adolescent Substance Use; Catherine Stanger and Hugh Garavan -- PART IV: EPILOGUE -- 17. How to Practically Apply Lessons Learned from Translational Neuroscience to Intervention Development: Ideas for the Road Ahead; Sarah W. Feldstein Ewing, Katie Witkiewitz, and Francesca M. Filbey. Subjects: MEDICAL/Neuroscience. MEDICAL/Evidence-Based Medicine. PSYCHOLOGY/Clinical Psychology. PSYCHOLOGY/Physiological Psychology. PSYCHOLOGY/Psychopatholo gy/Addiction. Drug addiction--Treatment. Human behavior. Dewey class no.: 362.29 Other class no.: MED057000 MED112000 PSY007000 PSY024000 PSY038000 Content type: text Media type: unmediated Carrier type: volume

Neurology: an evidence-based approach LCCN: 2011936746 Type of material: Book Main title: Neurology: an evidence-based approach/Jorge G. Burneo, Bart M. Demaerschalk, Mary E. Jenkins, editors.

Published/Produced: New York: Springer, [2012] ©2012 Description: xiv, 368 pages: color illustrations; 24 cm ISBN: 9780387885544 (acid-free paper) LC classification: RC346 .N45135 2012 Related names: Burneo, Jorge G., editor of compilation. Demaerschalk, Bart M., editor of compilation. Jenkins, Mary E., editor of compilation. Subjects: Neurology. Evidence-based medicine. Notes: Includes bibliographical references and index. Dewey class no.: 616.8 Invalid ISBN: 9780387885551 (ebook) Content type: text Media type: unmediated Carrier type: volume CALL NUMBER: RC346 .N45135 2012 Copy 1 Request in: Jefferson or Adams Building Reading Rooms

Neuropsychological assessment and intervention for youth: an evidence based approach to emotional and behavioral disorders LCCN: 2012030072 Type of material: Book Main title: Neuropsychological assessment and intervention for youth: an evidence based approach to emotional and behavioral disorders/edited by Linda A. Reddy, Adam S. Weissman, and James B. Hale. Edition: 1st ed. Published/Created: Washington, DC: American Psychological Association, c2013. Description: xiii, 364 p.; 26 cm. ISBN: 9781433812668 1433812665 LC classification: RJ499 .N426 2013 Related names: Reddy, Linda A. Weissman, Adam S. (Adam Scott), 1980- Hale, James B., 1961- American Psychological Association. Contents: Neuropsychological assessment and intervention for emotional and behavior disordered youth: opportunities for practice/Linda A. Reddy, Adam S. Weissman, and James B. Hale -- Anxiety disorders/Allison Waters, Lara J. Farrell, and Elizabeth Schilpzand -- Obsessive-compulsive disorder/Susanna W. Chang, Joseph O'Neill, and David Rosenberg -- Depressive disorders/Steven G. Feifer and Gurmal Rattan -- Bipolar disorder/Patricia D. Walshaw and Carrie E. Bearden -- Attention-deficit/hyperactivity disorder/James B. Hale ... [et al.] -- Attention-deficit/hyperactivity disorder predominantly inattentive type/Richard Gallagher and Jennifer Rosenblatt -- Conduct and oppositional defiant disorders/Jean Séguin and Mathieu Pilon -- Tourette's disorder and other tic disorders/Matt W. Specht and

Susanna W. Chang -- Mental retardation and other low-incidence disorders/Kathleen Armstrong, Jason Hangauer, and Heather Aggazi -- Pervasive developmental disorders/Justin J. Boseck, Elizabeth L. Roberds, and Andrew S. Davis -- Neurodevelopmental disorders and associated emotional/behavioral sequelae/Joanna Thome, Tina Drossos, and Scott J. Hunter -- Chronic pediatric medical conditions and comorbid psychopathology/Erin L. Steck-Silvestri ... [et al.] -- Understanding neuropsychopathology in the twenty-first century: current status, clinical application, and future directions/Leonard F. Koziol, Deborah E. Budding, and James B. Hale. Subjects: Mental Disorders--diagnosis. Adolescent. Brain--physiopathology. Child. Evidence-Based Medicine--methods. Mental Disorders--therapy. Notes: Includes bibliographical references and index. Dewey class no.: 616.800835 NLM class no.: WS 350 Other system no.: (DNLM)101592298 Shelf Location: FLM2014 029072 CALL NUMBER: RJ499 .N426 2013 OVERFLOWA5S Request in: Jefferson or Adams Building Reading Rooms (FLM1)

Nutrition in clinical practice: a comprehensive, evidence-based manual for the practitioner LCCN: 2014015290 Type of material: Book Personal name: Katz, David L., 1963- author. Main title: Nutrition in clinical practice: a comprehensive, evidence-based manual for the practitioner/David L. Katz, MD, MPH, FACPM, FACP, Director, Prevention Research Center, Yale University School of Public Health, Griffin Hospital, Clinical Instructor in Medicine, Yale University School of Medicine, Director, Integrative Medical Center, Griffin Hospital, President, American College of Lifestyle Medicine, Derby, Connecticut; with Rachel S.C. Friedman, MD, MHS, Department of Family Medicine, The Permanente Medical Group, Santa Rosa, California, Assistant Clinical Professor, Department of Community and Family Medicine, San Francisco, California, and Sean C. Lucan, MD, MPH, MS, Department of Family and Social Medicine, Albert Einstein College of Medicine, Montefiore Medical Center, Bronx, New York . Edition: Third edition. Published/Produced:

Philadelphia: Wolters Kluwer, [2015] ©2015 Description: xxi, 730 pages: illustrations; 26 cm. ISBN: 9781451186642 (paperback: alk. paper) 1451186649 (paperback: alk. paper) LC classification: RM216 .K37 2015 Related names: Friedman, Rachel S. C., author. Lucan, Sean C., author. Summary: "In nearly every level of treatment and counseling, care providers must take into account the effects of their patients' diets. Nutrition in Clinical Practice is written to guide health professionals in providing well-informed, compassionate, and effective dietary and weight-management counseling. This fully updated 3rd edition is edited by a leading authority in nutrition and preventive medicine. Practical and evidence-based, chapters address the effects of diet on health and a comprehensive array of illnesses, making it a vital and timely addition to any caregiver's library. Features: NEW data from hundreds of recent studies, NEW section: Contemporary Topics in Nutrition, Easy-reference format includes short chapters, links to current online articles, Contributors representing diverse expertise and practical experience with medical education, nutrition in clinical practice, and preventive medicine, Enhanced coverage of controversial topics, such as, the effects of sugar; health effects of obesity and the 'obesity paradox'; health effects of gluten and grains; nutritional therapy. Appendices includes ancillary materials such as clinically relevant formulas, nutrition data tables, and patient specific meal planners, all fully updated. Now with the print edition, enjoy the bundled interactive eBook edition, offering tablet, smartphone, or online access to: Complete content with enhanced navigation, A powerful search tool that pulls results from content in the book, your notes, and even the web, Cross-linked pages, references, and more for easy navigation, Highlighting tool for easier reference of key content throughout the text, Ability to take and share notes with friends and colleagues, Quick reference tabbing to save your favorite content for future use."-- Provided by publisher. Contents: Sect. I: Clinically relevant nutrient metabolism -- Clinically relevant carbohydrate metabolism -- Clinically relevant fat metabolism -- Clinically relevant protein metabolism -- Overview of clinically relevant micronutrient metabolism --

Sect. II: Nutritional management in clinical practice: diet, in sickness and in health -- Diet, weight regulation, and obesity -- Diet, diabetes mellitus, and insulin resistance -- Diet, atherosclerosis, and ischemic heart disease -- Diet and hypertension -- Diet and hemostasis -- Diet and cerebrovascular and peripheral vascular disease -- Diet and immunity -- Diet and cancer -- Diet and hematopoiesis: nutritional anesmias -- Diet, bone metabolism, and osteoporosis -- Diet and respiratory disease -- Diet and renal disease -- Diet and hepatobiliary disease -- Diet and common gastrointestional disorders -- Diet, dyspepsia, and peptic ulcer disease -- Diet and rheumatologic disease -- Diet and neurologic disorders -- Diet and dermatoses -- Diet and wound healing -- Food allergy and intolerance -- Eating disorders -- Malnutrition and cachexia -- Sect. III: Speical topics in clinical nutrition -- Diet, pregnancy, and lactation -- Diet and the menstrual cycle -- Diet and early development: pediatric nutrition -- Diet and adolescence -- Diet and senescence -- Ergogenic effects of foods and nutrients: diet and athletic performance & sports nutrition -- Endocrine effects of diet: phytoestrogens -- Diet, sleep-wake cycles, and mood -- Diet and cognitive function -- Diet and vision -- Diet and dentition -- Hunger, appetite, taste, and satiety -- Health effects of chocolate -- Health effects of ethanol -- Health effects of coffee -- Macronutrient food substitutes -- Vegetarianism, veganism, and macrobiotic diets -- Sect. IV: Diet and health promotion: establishing the theme of prudent nutrition -- Culture, evolutionary biology, and the determinants of dietary preference -- Dietary recommendations for health promotion and disease prevention -- Sect. V: Principles of effective dietary counseling -- Models of behavior modification for diet and activity patterns and weight management -- Dietary counseling in clinical practice -- Sect. VI: Controversies in contemporary clinical nutrition -- The calorie -- The search for scapegoats and silver bullets -- Obesity as disease. 505 0 $a Sect. VII: Appendices and resource materials -- Appendix A: Nutrition formulas of clinical interest -- Appendix B: Growth and body weight assessment tables -- Appendix C: Dietary intake assessment in the US population -- Appendix D: Dietary intake assessment instruments -- Appendix E: Nutrient/nutriceutical reference tables: intake range and dietary sources -- Appendix F: Resources for nutrient composition of foods -- Appendix G: Diet-drug interactions -- Appendix H: Nutrient remedies for common conditions: patient resources -- Appendix I: Print and web-based resource materials for professionals -- Appendix J: Print and web-based resource materials for patients -- Appendix K: Patient-specific meal planners -- Appendix L: Patient-specific supplement guidelines. Subjects: Nutritional Physiological Phenomena. Evidence-Based Medicine. Notes: Includes bibliographical references and index. Dewey class no.: 615.8/54 NLM class no.: QU 145 Other system no.: (DNLM)101630629 Content type: text Media type: unmediated Carrier type: volume CALL NUMBER: RM216 .K37 2015 Copy 1 Request in: Jefferson or Adams Building Reading Rooms 100. Evaluating obesity prevention efforts: A plan for measuring progress LCCN: 2012276159 Type of material: Book Main title: Evaluating obesity prevention efforts: A plan for measuring progress/Committee on Evaluating Progress of Obesity Prevention Efforts; Food and Nutrition Board; Lawrence W. Green, Leslie Sim, and Heather Breiner, editors. Published/Produced: Washington, D.C.: National Academies Press, [2013] Description: xi, 449 pages: illustrations (some color); 28 cm Links: National Academies http://www.nap.edu/catalog.php ?record_id=18334 ISBN: 0309285275 (pbk.) 9780309285278 (pbk.) LC classification: RA645.O23 E935 2013 Related names: Green, Lawrence W. editor. Sim, Leslie J. editor. Breiner, Heather, editor. Institute of Medicine (U.S.). Food and Nutrition Board. issuing body Summary: "Obesity poses one of the greatest public health challenges of the 21st century, creating serious health, economic, and social consequences for individuals and society. Despite acceleration in efforts to characterize, comprehend, and act on this problem, including implementation of preventive interventions, further understanding is needed on the progress and effectiveness of these interventions. Evaluating Obesity Prevention Efforts develops a concise and actionable plan for measuring the nation's progress in obesity prevention efforts--specifically, the success of policy and environmental strategies recommended in the 2012 IOM report Accelerating Progress in Obesity Prevention: Solving the Weight of the Nation. This book offers a framework that will provide guidance for systematic and routine planning, implementation, and evaluation of the advancement of obesity prevention efforts. This framework is for specific use with the goals and strategies from the 2012 report and can be used to assess the progress made in every community and throughout the country, with the ultimate goal of reducing the obesity epidemic. It offers potentially valuable guidance in improving the quality and effect of the actions being implemented. The recommendations of Evaluating Obesity Prevention Efforts focus on efforts to increase the likelihood that actions taken to prevent obesity will be evaluated, that their progress in accelerating the prevention of obesity will be monitored, and that the most promising practices will be widely disseminated."--Publisher's description. Contents: Improving the Usefulness of Obesity Evaluation Information to Potential Users -- Framework for Evaluation -- Indicators for the Evaluation Plans -- Evaluating Progress in Promoting Health Equity: A Review of Methods and Tools for Measurement -- National Obesity Evaluation Plan -- Community Obesity Assessment and Surveillance -- Monitoring and Summative Evaluation of Community Interventions -- Systems and Evaluation: Placing a Systems Approach in Context -- Taking Action: Recommendations for Evaluating Progress of Obesity Prevention Efforts -- Appendix A: Acronyms -- Appendix B: Glossary -- Appendix C: Guiding Principles for Evaluation -- Appendix D: Table of Indicator Data Sources -- Appendix E: Disparities Tables -- Appendix F: National Plan Resources -- Appendix G: Community Health Assessment and Surveillance Resources -- Appendix H: Community Intervention Resources -- Appendix I: Panel Agenda -- Appendix J: Committee Biographies. Subjects: Obesity--United States--Prevention--Evaluation. Evidence-based medicine. Obesity--Prevention.

Notes: Includes bibliographical references. Dewey class no.: 616.398 Other system no.: (OCoLC)ocn849593069 Content type: text Media type: unmediated Carrier type: volume Shelf Location: FLM2014 113124 CALL NUMBER: RA645.O23 E935 2013 OVERFLOWA5S Request in: Jefferson or Adams Building Reading Rooms (FLM1)

Observational studies in a learning health system: workshop Summary: LCCN: 2014397702 Type of material: Book Corporate name: Observational Studies in a Learning Health System (Workshop) (2013: Washington, D.C.) Main title: Observational studies in a learning health system: workshop summary/Claudia Grossmann and Joe Alper, rapporteurs; a Learning Health System Activity, Roundtable on Value & Science-Driven Health Care, Institute of Medicine of the National Academies. Published/Produced: Washington, D.C.: The National Academies Press, [2013] Description: xix, 114 pages: illustrations (chiefly color); 23 cm Links: National Academies Press http://www.nap.edu/catalog.php?record_id=18438 ISBN: 9780309290814 0309290813 LC classification: R850.A2 O27 2013 Related names: Grossmann, Claudia, 1978- author. Alper, Joe, author. Institute of Medicine (U.S.). Roundtable on Value & Science-Driven Health Care, issuing body. Patient-Centered Outcomes Research Institute (U.S.), sponsoring body. Summary: "Clinical research strains to keep up with the rapid and iterative evolution of medical interventions, clinical practice innovation, and the increasing demand for information on the clinical effectiveness of these advancements. In response to the growing availability of archived and real-time digital health data and the opportunities this data provides for research, as well as the increasing number of studies using prospectively collected clinical data, the Institute of Medicine's Roundtable on Value & Science-Driven Health Care convened a workshop on Observational Studies in a Learning Health System. Participants, including experts from a wide range of disciplines - clinical researchers, statisticians, biostatisticians, epidemiologists, health care informaticians, health care analytics, research funders, health products industry, clinicians, payers, and regulators - explored leading edge approaches to observational studies, charted a course for the use of the growing health data utility, and identified opportunities to advance progress. Workshop speakers and individual participants strove to identify stakeholder needs and barriers to the broader application of observational studies. Observational Studies in a Learning Health System is the summary of the workshop. This report explores the role of observational studies in the generation of evidence to guide clinical and health policy decisions. The report discusses concepts of rigorous observational study design and analysis, emerging statistical methods, and opportunities and challenges of observational studies to complement evidence from experimental methods, treatment heterogeneity, and effectiveness estimates tailored toward individual patients"--Publisher's description. Contents: Introduction -- Issues overview for observational studies in clinical research -- Engaging the issue of bias -- Generalizing randomized clinical trial results to broader populations -- Detecting treatment-effect heterogeneity -- Predicting individual responses -- Strategies going forward -- Common themes for progress. Subjects: Clinical medicine--Research--Congresses. Experimental design--Congresses. Evidence-based medicine--Congresses. Medical care--Congresses. Observational Study as Topic--methods. Research Design--standards. Prospective Studies. Data Collection--methods. Delivery of Health Care--methods. Evidence-Based Medicine--methods. Notes: "Observational Studies in a Learning Health System: an Institute of Medicine workshop, sponsored by the Patient-Centered Outcomes Research Institute; a Learning Health System Activity, IOM Roundtable on Value & Science-Driven Health Care, April 25-26, 2013, National Academy of Sciences"--Page 101. Includes bibliographical references. Dewey class no.: 610.72/4 Other system no.: (OCoLC)ocn867561314 Content type: text Media type: unmediated Carrier type: volume Shelf Location: FLM2015 028313 CALL NUMBER: R850.A2 O27 2013 OVERFLOWJ34 Request in: Jefferson or Adams Building Reading Rooms (FLM2)

Obstetric evidence based guidelines LCCN: 2011046454 Type of material: Book Main title: Obstetric evidence based guidelines/edited by Vincenzo Berghella. Edition: 2nd ed. Published/Created: New York: Informa Healthcare, c2012. Projected pub date: 1203 Description: p.; cm. ISBN: 9781841848242 (hb: alk. paper) Related names: Berghella, Vincenzo. Subjects: Pregnancy. Delivery, Obstetric--methods. Evidence-Based Medicine. Pregnancy Complications--prevention & control. Prenatal Care--methods. Notes: Includes bibliographical references and index. Series: Series in maternal-fetal medicine Series in maternal-fetal medicine. Dewey class no.: 618.2 NLM class no.: WQ 200 Other system no.: (DNLM)101572733

Ordinary medicine: extraordinary treatments, longer lives, and where to draw the line LCCN: 2014043465 Type of material: Book Personal name: Kaufman, Sharon R. Main title: Ordinary medicine: extraordinary treatments, longer lives, and where to draw the line/Sharon R. Kaufman. Published/Produced: Durham; London: Duke University Press, 2015. Projected pub date: 1505 Description: pages cm ISBN: 9780822359029 (hardcover: alk. paper) 9780822358886 (pbk.: alk. paper) 9780822375500 (e-book) LC classification: RA395.A3 K385 2015 Contents: Diagnosing Twenty-First-Century health care -- The quandary and unexamined ordinariness of Twenty-First-Century medicine -- Ordinary medicine in our aging society: the dilemma of longevity -- The chain of health care drivers -- The medical-industrial complex I: evidence-based medicine, the biomedical -- Economy, and the ascendance of clinical trials -- The medical-industrial complex II: access, industry, and the clinical trials -- Phenomenon -- "Reimbursement is critical for everything": medicare and the ethics of managing life -- Medicine's changing means and ends -- Standard and necessary treatments: the changing means and ends of technology -- Family matters: kidneys and new forms of care -- Influencing the character of the future: prognosis, risk, and time left -- For whose benefit? Our shared quandary -- Toward a new social contract?. Subjects: Medical care--United States. Medical ethics--United States. Medical care, Cost of--United States. Longevity--United States. Notes:

Includes bibliographical references and index. Series: Critical global health Critical global health. Dewey class no.: 362.10973 Geographic area code: n-us--- Content type: text Media type: unmediated Carrier type: volume

Orthopaedic basic science: foundations of clinical practice LCCN: 2012954830 Type of material: Book Main title: Orthopaedic basic science: foundations of clinical practice/edited by Regis J. O'Keefe, MD, PhD, professor and chair, associate dean for clinical affairs, Department of Orthopaedics, University of Rochester Medical Center, Rochester, New York, Constance R. Chu, MD, Albert B. Ferguson professor of orthopaedic surgery, professor of bioengineering, vice chair for translational research, director, Cartilage Restoration Center, Department of Orthopaedic Surgery, University of Pittsburgh, Pittsburgh, Pennsylvania, Joshua J. Jacobs, MD, William A. Hark, MD/Susanne G. Swift professor and chairman, Department of Orthopaedic Surgery, Rush University Medical Center, Chicago, Illinois, Thomas A. Einhorn, MD, chairman, Department of Orthopaedic Surgery, Boston University Medical Center, Boston, Massachusetts. Edition: Fouth edition. Published/Produced: Rosemont, IL: American Academy of Orthopaedic Surgeons, [2013] Description: xv, 544 pages: illustrations (some color); 28 cm ISBN: 9780892038435 0892038438 LC classification: RD731 .O75 2013 Related names: O'Keefe, Regis J., editor. Chu, Constance R., editor. Jacobs, Joshua J., 1956- editor. Einhorn, Thomas A., editor. American Academy of Orthopaedic Surgeons. Summary: The new, fourth edition developed in partnership with the Orthopaedic Research Society, is your concise and clinically relevant resource for the diagnosis and treatment of musculoskeletal diseases and conditions. This completely rewritten edition explains the functions and limitations of the science behind the decisions, treatments, and procedures you perform in your practice every day. Use it to build and reinforce your foundation of knowledge for applying advances in scientific discovery to your decision-making in the clinic and the OR. The new Clinical Science section covers ethics in research, evidence-based medicine, defining and using best-practice in orthopaedic decision-making, interpreting and evaluating clinical studies and more-- Source other than Library of Congress. Subjects: Orthopedics. Musculoskeletal system--Pathophysiology. Musculoskeletal Physiological Phenomena. Musculoskeletal Diseases. Musculoskeletal System--physiopathology. Orthopedic Procedures. Notes: "Developed with support from the Orthopaedic Research Society." "Bone and Joint Initiative, USA"--Page 4 cover. Includes bibliographical references and index. NLM class no.: WE 102 O77 2013 National bib agency no.: 101614539 Other system no.: (OCoLC)ocn835953167 Content type: text Media type: unmediated Carrier type: volume CALL NUMBER: RD731 .O75 2013 Copy 1 Request in: Jefferson or Adams Building Reading Rooms CALL NUMBER: RD731 .O75 2013 Copy 2 Request in: Reference - Science Reading Room (Adams, 5th Floor)

Palliative aspects in emergency care LCCN: 2012041603 Type of material: Book Main title: Palliative aspects in emergency care/edited by Paul L. DeSandre, Tammie E. Quest. Published/Created: Oxford: Oxford University Press, c2013. Description: xviii, 134 p.; 21 cm. ISBN: 9780199895618 (alk. paper) LC classification: R726.8 .P34255 2013 Related names: DeSandre, Paul L. Quest, Tammie E. Contents: Overview -- Trajectories and prognostication in emergency care -- Rapid palliative care assessment -- Cancer emergencies -- Malignant pain -- Non-malignant pain -- Symptom management -- Spiritual suffering and bereavement -- Communication -- Resuscitation, family presence, and last hours of living -- Hospice -- Legal and ethical issues of palliative care in the emergency. Subjects: Palliative Care. Emergency Service, Hospital. Evidence-Based Medicine. Hospice Care. Notes: Includes bibliographical references and index. Series: Oxford American palliative care library Oxford American palliative care library. Dewey class no.: 616.029 NLM class no.: WB 310 Other system no.: (DNLM)101593939

Perspectives on complementary and alternative medicines LCCN: 2012359173 Type of material: Book Main title: Perspectives on complementary and alternative medicines/editors, Ian Olver, Monica Robotin. Published/Created: London: Imperial College Press; Singapore: distributed by World Scientific Pub., c2012. Description: xxii, 465 p.: ill.; 24 cm. Links: http://site.ebrary.com/id/10529398 ebrary ISBN: 9781848165564 1848165560 LC classification: R733 .P4235 2012 Related names: Olver, Ian N. Robotin, Monica C. Subjects: Alternative medicine. Cancer--Alternative treatment. Integrative medicine. Evidence-based medicine. Complementary Therapies. Neoplasms--therapy. Integrative Medicine. Evidence-Based Medicine. Notes: Includes bibliographical references and index. Dewey class no.: 615.5 Other system no.: (OCoLC)ocn503042332 CALL NUMBER: R733 .P4235 2012 Copy 1 Request in: Jefferson or Adams Building Reading Rooms

Plumer's principles & practice of infusion therapy LCCN: 2013041203 Type of material: Book Personal name: Weinstein, Sharon, author. Uniform title: Plumer's principles & practice of intravenous therapy Main title: Plumer's principles & practice of infusion therapy/Sharon M. Weinstein, MS, RN, CRNI, FACW, FAAN, Mary E. Hagle, PhD, RN, FAAN. Edition: Ninth edition. Published/Produced: Philadelphia: Wolters Kluwer Health, [2014] Description: xxii, 830 pages: illustrations; 23 cm ISBN: 9781451188851 (pbk) LC classification: RM170 .W445 2014 Variant title: Plumer's principles and practice of infusion therapy Principles and practice of infusion therapy Related names: Hagle, Mary E., author. Contents: History of infusion therapy -- Minimizing risk and enhancing performance -- Nursing role and responsibilities -- Standards of practice -- Nurse and patient education -- Anatomy and physiology applied to infusion therapy -- Diagnostic testing and values -- Fluid and electrolyte balance -- Principles of parenteral administration -- Complications and nursing interventions -- Evidence-based infusion practice -- Infusion delivery systems and safety -- Peripheral venous access -- Central venous access -- Expanded approaches to access and monitoring -- Parenteral nutrition -- Blood and component therapy -- Pharmacology applied to infusion therapy -- Antineoplastic therapy -- Pain management -- Pediatric infusion therapy -- Infusion therapy in an older adult -- Infusion therapy across the continuum of care -- The future of infusion nursing: a global approach. Subjects: Infusions, Intravenous--methods. Infusions, Intravenous--nursing. Evidence-Based Medicine. Fluid Therapy--methods. Nurse's Role. Parenteral Nutrition--methods. Notes: Preceded by Plumer's principles & practice of intravenous therapy/Sharon M. Weinstein. 8th ed. c2007. Includes bibliographical references and index. Dewey class no.: 615/.6 NLM class no.: WB 354 Other system no.: (DNLM)101618275 Content type: text Media type: unmediated Carrier type: volume Shelf Location: FLM2015 013176 CALL NUMBER: RM170 .W445 2014 OVERFLOWJ34 Request in: Jefferson or Adams Building Reading Rooms (FLM2)

Point of care medicine LCCN: 2012040996 Type of material: Book Main title: Point of care medicine/[edited by] Anthony D. Slonim, Alexander B. Levitov, Paul Marik. Published/Created: New York: McGraw Hill Medical, c2013. Projected pub date: 1307 Description: p.; cm. ISBN: 9780071762984 (hardcover: alk. paper) 0071762981 (hardcover: alk. paper) Related names: Slonim, Anthony D. Levitov, Alexander. Marik, Paul Ellis. Contents: Bedside procedures/Christian H. Butcher -- Environmental emergencies/Colin G. Kaide, Hannah L. Hays, David P. Bahner -- Toxicology/Colin G. Kaide, Hannah L. Hays, David P. Bahner -- Cardiology/Alexander Levitov -- Endocrinology/David J. Castaldo, Jody P. Boggs -- Gastroenterology/Paul Marik -- Hematology/B. Mitchell Goodman III ... [et al.] -- Infectious diseases/Stephanie B. Troy ... [et al.] -- Nephrology/James S. Cain -- Neurology/Paul Marik -- Oncology/Shrirang Ajvalia, Shilpa Amara, Anthony D. Slonim -- Pulmonology/Himanshu Desai, Michael Hooper -- Rheumatology/Joan K. Kowalec, Robert G. Lahita -- Obstetrics/Allison R. Durica, Amanda B. Murchison, Patrice M. Weiss -- Gynecology/Amanda B. Murchison, Allison Durica, Patrice M. Weiss -- Perioperative care of the surgical patient/Ronald S. Chamberlain ... [et al.] -- Psychiatry/Nina

Khachiyants. Subjects: Point-of-Care Systems. Hospitalization. Evidence-Based Medicine. Form/Genre: Outlines. Notes: Includes bibliographical references and index. Dewey class no.: 362.11 NLM class no.: WX 162 Other system no.: (DNLM)101593757

Practical biostatistics: a user-friendly approach for evidence-based medicine LCCN: 2012474090 Type of material: Book Personal name: Suchmacher, Mendel. Main title: Practical biostatistics: a user-friendly approach for evidence-based medicine/Mendel Suchmacher, Mauro Geller. Edition: 1st ed. Published/Created: Amsterdam; Boston: Elsevier/Academic Press, 2012. Description: xii, 236 p.: ill.; 23 cm. ISBN: 9780124157941 0124157947 LC classification: QH323.5 .S83 2012 Cover title Practical biostatistics with Microsoft Excel Related names: Geller, Mauro. Subjects: Biometry. Medical statistics. Medicine--Research--Data processing. Biostatistics--methods. Evidence-Based Medicine. Notes: Includes bibliographical references and index. NLM class no.: 2012 H-094 WA 950 National bib agency no.: 101592022 016117128 Other system no.: (OCoLC)ocn793581624 Shelf Location: FLM2013 019799 CALL NUMBER: QH323.5 .S83 2012 OVERFLOWA5S Request in: Jefferson or Adams Building Reading Rooms (FLM1) CALL NUMBER: QH323.5 .S83 2012 LANDOVR Copy 2 Request in: Jefferson or Adams Building Reading Rooms - STORED OFFSITE

Practical clinical epidemiology for the veterinarian LCCN: 2014047527 Type of material: Book Personal name: Villarroel, Aurora, author. Main title: Practical clinical epidemiology for the veterinarian/Aurora Villarroel. Edition: First edition. Published/Produced: Ames, Iowa: John Wiley & Sons Inc., 2015. Projected pub date: 1505 Description: p.; cm. ISBN: 9781118472064 (pbk.) LC classification: SF780.9 .V55 2015 Contents: Describing health and disease -- Basic epidemiology concepts -- Evidence based medicine for the veterinarian -- Study designs -- Causation vs. association -- Diagnostic tests -- Outbreak investigations. Subjects: Veterinary epidemiology. Epidemiologic Methods--veterinary. Disease Outbreaks--veterinary. Evidence-Based

Practice. Notes: Includes bibliographical references and index. Additional formats: Online version: Villarroel, Aurora, author. Practical clinical epidemiology for the veterinarian First edition. Ames, Iowa: John Wiley & Sons Inc., 2015 9781118472040 (DLC) 2014048451 Dewey class no.: 636.089/44 NLM class no.: SF 780.9 Other system no.: (DNLM)101647792 Content type: text Media type: unmediated Carrier type: volume

Prevention of diabetes LCCN: 2013013319 Type of material: Book Main title: Prevention of diabetes/edited by Peter Schwarz, Prasuna Reddy. Published/Created: Chichester, West Sussex: John Wiley & Sons, 2013. Description: xii, 216 p.: ill.; 23 cm. ISBN: 9780470654651 (pbk.: alk. paper) 9781118661291 (ePDF) 9781118661307 (Mobi) 9781118661314 (ePub) 9781118661321 (oBook) LC classification: RC660.4 .P68 2013 Related names: Schwarz, Peter (Physician) Reddy, Prasuna. Contents: What have we learned from the number of clinical trials?/Jaana Lindström -- Identification of target populations for intervention/Paul Valensi and Emmanuel Cosson -- Diagnosis of prediabetes and diabetes prevention/Martin Buysschaert and Michael Bergman -- What do we know about recruitment and retention in diabetes prevention programs: an Australian perspective/Philip Vita ... [et al.] -- Depression and diabetes prevention/Norbert Hermanns -- Diabetes prevention in a challenging environment/Abdul Basit and Musarrat Riaz -- Prevention of diabetes and global migration/Bishwajit Bhowmik, Victoria Telle Hjellset, and Akhtar Hussain -- Diabetes prevention in practice: examples from the real world/Konstantinos Makrilakis ... [et al.] -- Quality management and outcome evaluation in diabetes prevention/Markku Peltonen and Rüdiger Landgraf -- Training of prevention managers/Peter Kronsbein -- Prevention of type 2 diabetes: the role of physical activity/Thomas Yates, Melanie Davies and Kamlesh Khunti -- Overview: potentials of new media for the training of health educators in the field of diabetes prevention/Daniel Tolks and Martin R. Fischer -- Practice approach for the implementation of diabetes prevention/Avivit Cahn, Baruch Itzhak and Itamar Raz. Subjects: Diabetes

Mellitus, Type 2--prevention & control. Diabetes Mellitus, Type 2--complications. Diabetes Mellitus, Type 2--diagnosis. Evidence-Based Medicine--education. Risk Factors. Notes: Includes bibliographical references and index. Dewey class no.: 616.4/62 NLM class no.: WK 810 Other system no.: (DNLM)101605284 Shelf Location: FLM2014 028085 CALL NUMBER: RC660.4 .P68 2013 OVERFLOWA5S Request in: Jefferson or Adams Building Reading Rooms (FLM1)

Prevention vs. treatment: what's the right balance? LCCN: 2011010087 Type of material: Book Main title: Prevention vs. treatment: what's the right balance?/edited by Halley S. Faust and Paul T. Menzel. Published/Created: Oxford: Apha Press, c2012. Description: xvi, 397 p.: ill.; 24 cm. ISBN: 9780199837373 (hc: alk. paper) LC classification: RA425 .P725 2012 Related names: Faust, Halley S. Menzel, Paul T., 1942- Contents: What is currently spent on prevention as compared to treatment?/Charles Roehrig ... [et al.] -- Prevention vs. cure: an economist's perspective on the right balance/Louise B. Russell -- Toward a more evidence-based preventive medicine: issues in the science of clinical prevention/Robert B. Wallace -- Prevention and the science and politics of evidence/Diana B. Petitti -- Historical perspectives on structural barriers to prevention/Halley S. Faust -- Our alleviation bias: why do we value alleviating harm more than preventing harm?/Halley S. Faust -- Treatment and prevention: what do we owe each other?/Norman Daniels -- The variable value of life and fairness to the already ill: two promising but tenuous arguments for treatment's priority/Paul T. Menzel -- The slow transition of U.S. law toward a greater emphasis on prevention/Thaddeus Mason Pope -- Should the value of future health benefits be time-discounted?/Paul T. Menzel -- Prevention vs. treatment: how do we allocate scarce resources from Jewish ethical perspectives?/Alan Jotkowitz and Shimon Glick -- Cure vs. prevention: Catholic perspectives/Nuala Kenny -- Loving God and the neighbor: Protestant insights for prevention and treatment/Ana Marie Vigen -- Apocalypse and health: treatment and prevention in the Seventh-day Adventist tradition/Roy Branson --

Prevention vs. treatment in Hong Kong: constrained utilitarianism with a Chinese character/Ho Mun Chan. Subjects: Medicine, Preventive--United States. Preventive health services--United States. Evidence-based medicine--United States. Preventive Health Services--United States. Evidence-Based Medicine--United States. Health Promotion--United States. Primary Prevention--United States. Religion and Medicine--United States. Therapeutics--United States. Notes: Includes bibliographical references and index. Dewey class no.: 614.4/40973 Geographic area code: n-us--- NLM class no.: WA 108 Other system no.: (DNLM)101555738 Shelf Location: FLM2014 178901 CALL NUMBER: RA425 .P725 2012 OVERFLOWA5S Request in: Jefferson or Adams Building Reading Rooms (FLM1)

Principles and practice of child neurology in infancy LCCN: 2012540966 Type of material: Book Main title: Principles and practice of child neurology in infancy/edited by Colin Kennedy, Professor of Neurology and Paediatrics, Clinical Neurosciences, University of Southampton, and Honorary Consultant, Paediatric Neurologist, Southampton University Hospital NHS Foundation Trust, Southampton, United Kingdom. Published/Produced: London: Mac Keith Press, 2012. Description: xvi, 374 pages: illustrations (some color); 24 cm ISBN: 9781908316356 1908316357 LC classification: RJ486 .P75 2012 Related names: Kennedy, Colin, editor. Contents: Terms, definitions and concepts/Colin Kennedy -- Interprofessional working: user and carer involvement/Audrone Prasauskiene and Maryze Schoneveld van der Linde -- Clinical epidemiology and evidence-based medicine/Andrew L. Lux -- Promoting child development/Boika Rechel and Dainius Puras -- Neurological and neurodevelopmental assessment/Leena Haataja, Vittorio Belmonti and Giovanni Cioni -- Prevention of neurological disease in infants/Jane Williams and Colin Kennedy -- Cranial imaging/Brigitte Vollmer -- Neurophysiological investigations/Bernhard Schmitt and Varsine Jaladyan -- Biochemical and haematological testing -- Valerie Walker and Mary Morgan -- Drug treatments: drugs, vitamins and minerals/Imti Choonara and Peter Baxter -- Nonpharmacological treatment/Ilona Autti-Rämö -- Neonatal encephalopathy/Gian Paolo Chiaffoni and Daniele Trevisanuto -- Neonatal seizures, including metabolic epileptic encephalopathies/Barbara Plecko -- Acute non-febrile encephalopathy/Tiina Talvik, Fenella Kirkham, Tuuli Metsvaht and Inga Talvik -- Acute neurological illness with fever: meningitis, encephalitis and infective space-occupying lesions/Rachel Kneen and Charles Newton -- Post-neonatal epileptic seizures/Hans Hartmann and J. Helen Cross -- Non-epileptic paroxysmal disorders in infancy/John B.P. Stephenson and Alla Nechay -- Macrocephaly, including hydrocephalus/Colin Kennedy -- Microcephaly, including congenital infections/Richard Chin and Vlatka Mejaski-Bosnjak -- The floppy infant/Ulrika Ådén and Thomas Sejersen -- Early developmental impairment and neurological abnormalities at birth/Richard W. Newton, Ilona Autti- Rämö and Audrone Prasauskiene -- Cerebral palsy/Florian Heinen and Peter Baxter -- Central nervous system disorders of movement other than cerebral palsy/Peter Baxter and Florian Heinen -- Progressive loss of skills/Meral Topcu, Dilek Yalnýzoglu and Richard Newton. Subjects: Pediatric neurology. Nervous System Diseases. Infant. Pediatric neurology. Notes: Includes bibliographical references and index. NLM class no.: 2013 D-819 WS 340 National bib agency no.: 101607577 Other system no.: (OCoLC)ocn823751491 Content type: text Media type: unmediated Carrier type: volume CALL NUMBER: RJ486 .P75 2012 Copy 1 Request in: Jefferson or Adams Building Reading Rooms

Principles and techniques of trauma-centered psychotherapy LCCN: 2015006560 Type of material: Book Main title: Principles and techniques of trauma-centered psychotherapy/edited by David Read Johnson, Hadar Lubin. Edition: First edition. Published/Produced: Washington, DC: American Psychiatric Publishing, [2015] Projected pub date: 1505 Description: p.; cm. ISBN: 9781585625147 (pbk.: alk. paper) LC classification: RC480 Related names: Johnson, David Read, editor. Lubin, Hadar, editor. American Psychiatric Publishing, publisher. Contents: The developing cultural context of trauma-centered psychotherapy -- Axioms of trauma-centered psychotherapy -- Establishing the trauma-centered frame -- Principles of trauma-centered psychotherapy -- The four main techniques -- The first session -- Continuing the trauma history: getting the details and formulating the trauma schemas-- Conducting ongoing treatment: processing the trauma schemas in current behavior -- The gap: when the trauma schemas emerge in the therapeutic relationship -- Long term process in trauma-centered treatment -- Handling the edges -- Working with dissociative identity disordered clients -- Working with borderline personality disordered clients -- Trauma-centered group psychotherapy -- Trauma-centered couples and family psychotherapy -- Adjunctive methods -- Strains on the therapist -- Limits to the trauma centered approach. Subjects: Stress Disorders, Post-Traumatic--therapy. Evidence-Based Medicine. Psychotherapy--methods. Notes: Includes bibliographical references and index. Dewey class no.: 616.89/14 NLM class no.: WM 172.5 Other system no.: (DNLM)101651972 Content type: text Media type: unmediated Carrier type: volume

Principles of research design and drug literature evaluation LCCN: 2013050973 Type of material: Book Main title: Principles of research design and drug literature evaluation/edited by Rajender R. Aparasu, MPharm, PhD, FAPhA, Professor and Chair, Department of Pharmaceutical Health Outcomes and Policy, College of Pharmacy, University of Houston, Houston, Texas, John P. Bentley, RPh, PhD, FAPhA, Professor of Pharmacy Administration, Research Professor in the Research Institute of Pharmaceutical Sciences, School of Pharmacy, University of Mississippi, Oxford, Mississippi. Published/Produced: Burlington, MA: Jones & Bartlett Learning, [2015] ©2015 Description: xxx, 370 pages: illustrations; 26 cm ISBN: 9781449691301 (pbk.) 1449691307 (pbk.) 9781284038798 (with online access code) 1284038793 (with online access code) LC classification: RM301.25 .P754 2015 Related names: Aparasu, Rajender R., editor of compilation. Bentley, John P.

(John Paul), 1970- editor of compilation. Contents: The scientific approach to research and practice -- Ethical considerations in clinical research -- Research design and methods -- Randomized controlled trials -- Cohort and case control studies -- Other observational studies -- Case reports and case series -- Measurement and descriptive analysis -- Interpretation and basic statistical concepts -- Bivariate analysis and comparing groups -- Simple and multiple linear regression -- Logistic regression and survival analysis -- Sample size and power analysis -- Systematic review and meta-analysis -- Principles of evidence-based medicine -- Introduction to drug literature -- Evaluating clinical literature: an overview -- Evaluating randomized clinical trials -- Evaluating observational studies -- Applying drug literature to patient care -- Basics of journal club. Subjects: Drugs--Research. Drugs--Research--Statistical methods. Evidence-based medicine. Pharmacology. Pharmacology. Research Design. Statistics as Topic. Notes: Includes bibliographical references and index. Dewey class no.: 615.1072/4 NLM class no.: QV 20.5 Other system no.: (DNLM)101622591 Content type: text Media type: unmediated Carrier type: volume Shelf Location: FLM2015 048810 CALL NUMBER: RM301.25 .P754 2015 OVERFLOWJ34 Request in: Jefferson or Adams Building Reading Rooms (FLM2)

Professional development, reflection, and decision-making in nursing and health care LCCN: 2013003060 Type of material: Book Main title: Professional development, reflection, and decision-making in nursing and health care/edited by Melanie Jasper, Megan Rosser, Gail Mooney; with contributions from Georgina Koubel and Paul Elliott. Edition: 2nd ed. Published/Created: Chichester, West Sussex; Hoboken, New Jersey: Wiley-Blackwell, 2013. Description: viii, 245 p.: ill.; 25 cm. ISBN: 9780470658383 (softback: alk. paper) 9781118303252 (eMobi) 9781118303269 (ePDF) 9781118303276 (ePub) LC classification: RT42 .J37 2013 Related names: Jasper, Melanie. Rosser, Megan. Mooney, Gail P. Jasper, Melanie. Professional development, reflection, and decision-making. Contents: The context of professional development/Melanie Jasper and Gail Mooney -- Reflection and reflective practice/Melanie Jasper and Megan Rosser -- Reflective writing for professional development/Melanie Jasper and Gail Mooney -- Decision-making in professional practice/Georgina Koubel -- Work-based learning and portfolios/Melanie Jasper and Megan Rosser -- Moving from clinical supervision to person-centred development (PCD): a paradigm shift/Paul Elliott -- Practising as a professional/Melanie Jasper and Megan Rosser. Subjects: Nursing. Decision Making. Evidence-Based Medicine. Nursing Theory. Notes: Rev. ed. of: Professional development, reflection, and decision-making/Melanie Jasper. 2006. Includes bibliographical references and index. Dewey class no.: 610.73 NLM class no.: WY 16.1 Other system no.: (DNLM)101600522 Shelf Location: FLM2014 032128 CALL NUMBER: RT42 .J37 2013 OVERFLOWA5S Request in: Jefferson or Adams Building Reading Rooms (FLM1)

Protocols for high-risk pregnancies: an evidence-based approach LCCN: 2015003151 Type of material: Book Main title: Protocols for high-risk pregnancies: an evidence-based approach/edited by John T. Queenan, Catherine Y. Spong, Charles J. Lockwood. Edition: Sixth edition. Published/Produced: Chichester, West Sussex; Hoboken, NJ: John Wiley and Sons, Inc., 2015. Projected pub date: 1506 Description: p.; cm. ISBN: 9781119000877 (cloth) LC classification: RG571 Related names: Queenan, John T., editor. Spong, Catherine Y., editor. Lockwood, Charles J., editor. Subjects: Pregnancy Complications. Pregnancy, High-Risk. Evidence-Based Medicine. Notes: Includes bibliographical references and index. Additional formats: Online version: Protocols for high-risk pregnancies Sixth edition. Chichester, West Sussex; Hoboken, NJ: John Wiley and Sons, Inc., 2015 9781119001249 (DLC) 2015003591 Dewey class no.: 618.3 NLM class no.: WQ 240 Other system no.: (DNLM)101650193 Content type: text Media type: unmediated Carrier type: volume

Psychodynamic psychotherapy research: evidence-based practice and practice-based evidence LCCN: 2011943750 Type of material: Book Main title: Psychodynamic psychotherapy research: evidence-based practice and practice-based evidence/Raymond A. Levy, J. Stuart Ablon, Horst Kächele, editors; foreword by Robert J. Waldinger. Published/Created: New York: Humana Press, c2012. Description: xxxiii, 646 p.: ill.; 26 cm. ISBN: 9781607617914 (hbk: alk. paper) 1607617919 (hbk: alk. paper) 9781607617921 (e-ISBN) 1607617927 (e-ISBN) LC classification: RC489.P72 P788 2012 Related names: Levy, Raymond A. Ablon, J. Stuart. Kächele, Horst, 1944- Subjects: Psychodynamic psychotherapy. Psychodynamic psychotherapy--Research. Evidence-based psychiatry. Psychoanalytic Therapy. Evidence-Based Medicine. Research. Notes: Includes bibliographical references and index. Series: Current clinical psychiatry Current clinical psychiatry. Dewey class no.: 616.89/14 NLM class no.: 2012 H-831 WM 460.6 National bib no.: GBB0E2951 National bib agency no.: 101593850 Other system no.: (OCoLC)ocn775397847 Shelf Location: FLM2013 001629 CALL NUMBER: RC489.P72 P788 2012 OVERFLOWA5S Request in: Jefferson or Adams Building Reading Rooms (FLM1)

Quality management and managerialism in healthcare: a critical historical survey LCCN: 2014024812 Type of material: Book Personal name: Beck, Matthias, 1964-, author. Main title: Quality management and managerialism in healthcare: a critical historical survey/Matthias Beck, Sara Melo. Published/Produced: Basingstoke, Hampshire; New York, NY: Palgrave Macmillan, 2014. Projected pub date: 1410 Description: p.; cm. ISBN: 9781137351982 (hardback) LC classification: RA399.A3 Related names: Melo, Sara, author. Summary: "Quality Management and Managerialism in Healthcare creates a comprehensive and systematic international survey of various perspectives on healthcare quality management together with some of their most pertinent critiques. Chapter one starts with a general discussion of the factors that drove the introduction of management paradigms into public sector and health management contexts in the mid to late 1980s. Chapter two explores the rise of risk awareness in medicine; which, prior to the 1980s, stood largely in isolation to the implementation of managerial performance targets. Chapter three investigates the widespread adoption of performance management and clinical governance frameworks during the 1980s and 1990s. This is followed by Chapters four and five which examine systems based models of patient safety and the evidence-based medicine movement as exemplars of managerial perspectives on healthcare quality. Chapter six discusses potential future avenues for the development of alternative perspectives on quality of care which emphasise workforce involvement. The book concludes by reviewing the factors which have underpinned the managerialist trajectory of healthcare management over the past decades and explores the potential impact of nascent technologies such as 'connected health' and 'telehealth' on future developments"--Provided by publisher. Contents: Machine generated contents note: -- 1. Managerialism: A Historical Overview 2. Risk in Medicine: Early Developments to the 1980s 3. Quality Management in Health care 4. Models of Patient Safety and Critique 5. Evidence-based Medicine 6. Managerialism in Healthcare: Future Avenues. Subjects: Quality Assurance, Health Care--history. History, 20th Century. History, 21st Century. Quality Assurance, Health Care--methods. Dewey class no.: 362.1068 NLM class no.: W 84.41 Other system no.: (DNLM)101635800 Content type: text Media type: unmediated Carrier type: volume

Queenan's management of high-risk pregnancy: an evidence-based approach LCCN: 2011027303 Type of material: Book Main title: Queenan's management of high-risk pregnancy: an evidence-based approach/edited by John T. Queenan, Catherine Y. Spong, Charles J. Lockwood. Edition: 6th ed. Published/Created: Chichester, West Sussex: Wiley-Blackwell, 2012. Projected pub date: 1203 Description: p.; cm. ISBN: 9780470655764 (hard cover: alk. paper) 0470655763 (hard cover: alk. paper) LC classification: RG571 .M24 2012 Variant title: Management of high-risk pregnancy Related titles: Management of high-risk pregnancy. Related names: Queenan, John T. Spong, Catherine Y. Lockwood, Charles

J. Subjects: Pregnancy--Complications. Pregnancy Complications. Evidence-Based Medicine. Pregnancy, High-Risk. Notes: Rev. ed. of: Management of high-risk pregnancy/edited by John T. Queenan, Catherine Y. Spong, Charles J. Lockwood. 5th. 2007. Includes bibliographical references and index. Dewey class no.: 618.3 NLM class no.: WQ 240 Other system no.: (DNLM)101563576

Recurrent pregnancy loss: causes, controversies, and treatment LCCN: 2015000795 Type of material: Book Uniform title: Recurrent pregnancy loss (Carp) Main title: Recurrent pregnancy loss: causes, controversies, and treatment/edited by Howard J. A. Carp, MB, BS, FRCOG, Clinical Professor, Obstetrics and Gynecology, Sheba Medical Center, Tel Hashomer, Israel and Sackler School of Medicine, Tel Aviv University, Israel. . Edition: Second edition. Published/Produced: Boca Raton: CRC Press, Taylor & Francis Group, 2015. Description: xvii, 438 pages: illustrations; 27 cm. ISBN: 9781482216141 (hardcover: alk. paper) 1482216140 (hardcover: alk. paper) LC classification: RG648 .R37 2015 Related names: Carp, Howard J. A., editor. Summary: "Recurrent pregnancy loss presents a vexing clinical problem primarily for medical professionals treating patients in reproductive medicine and in maternal-fetal medicine. However, with its numerous causes and various suggested treatment options, the problem is more multidisciplinary in nature, involving gynecology, genetics, endocrinology, immunology, pediatrics, and internal medicine. Exploring basic science and clinical applications, the second edition of the bestselling text . Recurrent Pregnancy Loss: Causes, Controversies, and Treatment provides an authoritative and comprehensive update on advances in the understanding and management of this troubling phenomenon.The book covers basic scientific topics such as genetics and cytokines and profiles major advances in immunology, endocrinology, and thrombotic mechanism. It discusses the methodology of clinical research and the application of evidence-based medicine to clinical practice. It also reviews various late obstetric complications, along with issues caused by extreme prematurity and possible resulting handicaps. This second edition presents new material on the latest controversies, featuring opinions from both sides of ongoing debates. It includes new chapters on autoimmunity, third party reproduction, the use of immunostimulants such as CSF, and Chinese medicine.Designed for specialists working in reproductive medicine clinics and those involved with maternal-fetal care, the book is also ideal for generalists and gynaecologists seeking a comprehensive view of developments in the field"--Provided by publisher. Subjects: Fetal death. Abortion, Habitual. Notes: Includes bibliographical references and index. Series: Series in maternal-fetal medicine Series in maternal-fetal medicine. 2158-0855 Dewey class no.: 618.3/92 NLM class no.: WQ 225 Other system no.: (DNLM)101649127 Content type: text Media type: unmediated Carrier type: volume Shelf Location: FLM2015 060253 CALL NUMBER: RG648 .R37 2015 OVERFLOWJ34 Request in: Jefferson or Adams Building Reading Rooms (FLM2)

Research methods in health: foundations for evidence-based practice LCCN: 2013427219 Type of material: Book Uniform title: Research methods in health (Liamputtong) Main title: Research methods in health: foundations for evidence-based practice/edited by Pranee Liamputtong. Edition: Second edition. Published/Produced: South Melbourne, Victoria, Australia: Oxford University Press, 2013. ©2013 Description: xxxv 521 pages: illustrations; 28 cm. ISBN: 9780195520064 (paperback) 0195520068 (paperback) LC classification: RA440.85 .R463 2013 Related names: Liamputtong, Pranee, 1955- editor. Subjects: Health--Research--Methodology. Medical care--Research--Methodology. Evidence-based medicine. Health Services Research--methods. Evidence-Based Medicine. Research Design. Medical care--Research--Methodology. Public health--Research--Methodology. Notes: Includes bibliographical references (pages 466-509) and index. Dewey class no.: 362.1072 NLM class no.: 2014 C-775 W 84.3 National bib no.: GBB347043 National bib agency no.: 101625248 016385112 Other system no.: (OCoLC)ocn843807740 Content type: text Media type: unmediated Carrier type: volume

Shelf Location: FLM2015 059812 CALL NUMBER: RA440.85 .R463 2013 OVERFLOWJ34 Request in: Jefferson or Adams Building Reading Rooms (FLM2)

Review of NASA's Evidence Reports on Human Health Risks: 2013 letter report LCCN: 2014498659 Type of material: Book Corporate name: Institute of Medicine (U.S.). Committee to Review NASA's Evidence Reports on Human Health Risks, author. Main title: Review of NASA's Evidence Reports on Human Health Risks: 2013 letter report/Committee to Review NASA's Evidence Reports on Human Health Risks, Board on Health Sciences Policy; Carol E.H. Scott-Conner, Daniel R. Masys, Catharyn T. Liverman, and Margaret A. McCoy, editors; Institute of Medicine of the National Academies. Published/Produced: Washington, D.C.: The National Academies Press, [2014] ©2014 Description: ix, 51 pages; 23 cm Links: http://www.ncbi.nlm.nih.gov/books/NBK217927/ National Academies Press http://www.nap.edu/catalog.php?record_id=18575 ISBN: 9780309296526 0309296528 LC classification: RC1135 .I58 2014 Related names: Scott-Conner, Carol E. H., editor. Masys, Daniel, editor. Liverman, Catharyn T., editor. McCoy, Margaret A., editor. Institute of Medicine (U.S.), publisher. Summary: "Review of NASA's Evidence Reports on Human Health Risks: 2013 Letter Report is the first in a series of five reports from the Institute of Medicine that will independently review more than 30 evidence reports that thc National Aeronautics and Space Administration has compiled on human health risks for long-duration and exploration space flights. This report builds on the 2008 IOM report Review of NASA's Human Research Program Evidence Books: A Letter Report, which provided an initial and brief review of the evidence reports. This letter report reviews three evidence reports and examines the quality of the evidence, analysis, and overall construction of each report; identifies existing gaps in report content; and provides suggestions for additional sources of expert input. The report analyzes each evidence report's overall quality, which included readability; internal consistency; the source and breadth of cited evidence; identification of existing knowledge and research gaps; authorship expertise; and, if applicable, response to recommendations from the 2008 IOM letter report."--Publisher's description. Contents: Review of NASA's Evidence Reports on Human Health Risks: 2013 letter report -- Appendix A: Meeting Agendas -- Appendix B: Committee Bio-sketches. Subjects: United States. National Aeronautics and Space Administration. United States. National Aeronautics and Space Administration. United States. National Aeronautics and Space Administration. Space medicine. Evidence-based medicine. Aerospace Medicine. Space Flight. Evidence-Based Medicine. Risk Assessment. Evidence-based medicine. Space medicine. Notes: Includes bibliographical references (pages 35-40). Additional formats: Also issued online. Dewey class no.: 616.9/80214 Geographic area code: n-us--- NLM class no.: 2014 G-780 WD 751 National bib agency no.: 101634869 Other system no.: (OCoLC)ocn874098496 Content type: text Media type: unmediated Carrier type: volume CALL NUMBER: RC1135 .I58 2014 Copy 1 Request in: Jefferson or Adams Building Reading Rooms

Scientific basis of healthcare. Angina LCCN: 2011038877 Type of material: Book Main title: Scientific basis of healthcare. Angina/editors, Colin R. Martin, Victor R. Preedy. Edition: 1st ed. Published/Created: Boca Raton, FL: CRC Press/Taylor & Francis Group; Enfield, N.H: Science Publishers, c2012. Description: x, 212 p.: ill. (some col.); 24 cm. ISBN: 9781578087327 (hardcover: alk. paper) LC classification: RC685.A6 S34 2012 Variant title: Angina Related names: Martin, Colin R., 1964- Preedy, Victor R. Contents: Epidemiology of angina/John F. Beltrame -- Chest pain: cardiac and non-cardiac causes/Geraldine Lee -- Coronary plaque rupture in patients with acute coronary syndrome/Toshio Imanishi -- The use and application of angina questionnaires/Norul Badriah Hassan and Muhammad Termizi Hassan -- American College of Cardiology/American Heart Association guidelines for ST-elevation myocardial infarction: overview of guidelines for care before, during, and after STEMI/Rohit S. Loomba and Rohit R. Arora -- Non-invasive coronary angiography with cardiac CT in patients with angina pectoris/Christof Burgstahler, Harald Brodoefel, and Stephen Schroeder -- Drugs used in angina: an overview/Mario Marzilli and Alda Huqi -- Current clinical application of direct thrombin inhibitors in angina pectoris/Bernardo Cortese and Marco Centola -- Anti-anginal drugs in focus: trimetazidine/Mario Marzilli and Alda Huqi -- Enhanced external counterpulsation therapy in coronary artery disease management/Ozlem Soran and Debra L. Braverman. Subjects: Angina Pectoris. Evidence-Based Medicine--methods. Myocardial Infarction. Notes: Includes bibliographical references and index. Dewey class no.: 362.196/122 NLM class no.: WG 298 Other system no.: (DNLM)101569384 Shelf Location: FLM2014 151472 CALL NUMBER: RC685.A6 S34 2012 OVERFLOWA5S Request in: Jefferson or Adams Building Reading Rooms (FLM1)

Shadow medicine: the placebo in conventional and alternative therapies LCCN: 2013048051 Type of material: Book Personal name: Haller, John S., Jr., 1940- author. Main title: Shadow medicine: the placebo in conventional and alternative therapies/John S. Haller Jr. Published/Produced: New York: Columbia University Press, [2014] ©2014 Description: xxix, 255 pages; 24 cm ISBN: 9780231169042 (cloth: alk. paper) 0231169043 (cloth: alk. paper) LC classification: R733 .H35 2014 Variant title: Placebo in conventional and unconventional therapies Contents: Evidence-based medicine -- Postmodernist medicine -- The powerful placebo -- Politics of healing -- Complementary and alternative medicine's challenge: a case study -- Reassessment. Subjects: Alternative medicine. Placebos (Medicine) Placebos. Complementary Therapies. Evidence-Based Medicine. Placebo Effect. Notes: Includes bibliographical references (pages 215-242) and index. Dewey class no.: 615.5 NLM class no.: WB 330 Other system no.: (DNLM)101621286 Invalid ISBN: 9780231537704 (ebook) Content type: text Media type: unmediated Carrier type: volume Shelf Location: FLM2015 062907 CALL NUMBER: R733 .H35 2014 OVERFLOWJ34 Request in: Jefferson or Adams Building Reading Rooms (FLM2)

Small animal soft tissue surgery LCCN: 2012005065 Type of material: Book Main title: Small animal soft tissue surgery/edited by Eric Monnet. Published/Created: Ames, Iowa: John Wiley & Sons, 2013. Description: xx, 849 p.: $b ill. (some col.); 29 cm. + 1 DVD-ROM (4 3/4 in.) ISBN: 9780813807829 (hardcover: alk. paper) 0813807824 (hardcover: alk. paper) LC classification: SF981 .S64 2013 Related names: Monnet, Eric. Summary: "Small Animal Soft Tissue Surgery is a comprehensive, in-depth resource for well-referenced, current information on small animal soft tissue surgery. Offering detailed surgical techniques in a well-illustrated, easy-to-follow format, the book covers the full range of surgically treated diseases and syndromes, with video clips and slideshows to demonstrate surgical procedures on an accompanying DVD. Small Animal Soft Tissue Surgery presents the state of the art for surgical conditions encountered in small animal surgery. Divided into chapters by body system, each section will begin with a brief review of the anatomy and physiology, with pathophysiology, diagnosis, treatment, and prognosis described in detail. Illustrations accompany the description of surgical techniques, and some discussion of evidence-based medicine is incorporated throughout. Small Animal Soft Tissue Surgery is an essential reference for small animal surgeons, residents, and practitioners performing soft tissue surgery"--Provided by publisher. Subjects: Pet medicine. Veterinary surgery. Soft tissue injuries--Surgery. Soft Tissue Injuries--veterinary. Surgery, Veterinary--methods. Pets--surgery. Notes: Includes bibliographical references and index. Dewey class no.: 636.089/7 NLM class no.: SF 914.3 Other system no.: (DNLM)101577676 CALL NUMBER: SF981 .S64 2013 Copy 1 Request in: See Reference Staff. By Appt in Jefferson Main RR (MRC)

Smith's patient-centered interviewing: an evidence-based method LCCN: 2011041384 Type of material: Book Main title: Smith's patient-centered interviewing: an evidence-based method/Auguste H. Fortin ... [et al.]. Edition: 3rd ed. Published/Created: New York: McGraw-Hill Professional, 2012. Projected pub date: 1204 Description: p.; cm. ISBN:

9780071760003 (pbk.) Variant title: Patient-centered interviewing Related names: Fortin, Auguste H. Smith, Robert C. (Robert Charles), 1937- Patient-centered interviewing. Summary: "A unique introductory guide to the principles of patient communication in clinical medicine, Patient Centered Interviewing: An Evidence-Based Method, is a practical introductory textbook covering the essentials of the patient interview. Teaching the renowned 5-Step Methodology, the book covers all the principles of conducting an effective patient interview, from the basics of interviewing to advanced situations in patient encounters. Featuring carefully screened data and results from research, this is the most evidence-based textbook on the subject. Pedagogy includes learning and practice exercises in each chapter"--Provided by publisher. Contents: Machine generated contents note: 1. Interviewing 2. Facilitating Skills 3. Patient-Centered Interviewing 4. Symptom-Defining Skills 5. Doctor-Centered Interviewing 6. Advanced Interviewing: Adapting the Interview to Different Situations and Other Practical Issues 7. Advanced Interviewing: The Provider-Patient Relationship 8. Summarizing and Presenting the Patient's Story 9. Patient EducationAppendix A. Research Report from the Annals of Internal Medicine: Academia and Clinic Appendix B. Foreword to the First Edition Appendix C. Examples of Emotions Appendix D. Complete Write-Up of Mrs. Jones' Initial Evaluation Subject Index. Subjects: Medical History Taking--methods. Evidence-Based Medicine. Physician-Patient Relations. Notes: Rev. ed. of: Patient-centered interviewing: an evidence-based method/Robert C. Smith. 2nd ed. c2002. Includes bibliographical references and index. Dewey class no.: 616.07/51 NLM class no.: WB 290 Other system no.: (DNLM)101570472

Statistical methods for dynamic treatment regimes: reinforcement learning, causal inference, and personalized medicine LCCN: 2013939595 Type of material: Book Personal name: Chakraborty, Bibhas, author. Main title: Statistical methods for dynamic treatment regimes: reinforcement learning, causal inference, and personalized medicine/Bibhas

Chakraborty, Erica E.M. Moodie. Published/Produced: New York, NY: Springer, [2013] ©2013 Description: xvi, 204 pages: illustrations (some color); 24 cm ISBN: 9781461474272 (alk. paper) 1461474272 (alk. paper) LC classification: RA409 .C42 2013 Related names: Moodie, Erica E. M., author. Summary: Presents statistical methods developed to address questions of estimation and inference for dynamic treatment regimes, a branch of personalized medicine. These methods are demonstrated with their conceptual underpinnings and illustration through analysis of real and simulated data, and their application to the practice of personalized medicine, which emphasizes the systematic use of individual patient information to optimize patient health care. Provides an overview of methodology and results gathered from journals, proceedings, and technical reports with the goal of orienting researchers to the field. Readers need familiarity with elementary calculus, linear algebra, and basic large-sample theory to use this text. Throughout the text, authors direct readers to available code or packages in different statistical languages to facilitate implementation. In cases where code does not already exist, the authors provide analytic approaches in sufficient detail that any researcher with knowledge of statistical programming could implement the methods from scratch. Applicable to a wide range of researchers, including statisticians, epidemiologists, medical researchers, and machine learning researchers interested in medical applications, as well as advanced graduate students in statistics and biostatistics -- Source other than Library of Congress. Contents: Introduction -- The data: observational studies and sequentially randomized trials -- Statistical reinforcement learning -- Semi-parametric estimation of optimal DTRs by modeling contrasts of conditional mean outcomes -- Estimation of optimal DTRs by directly modeling regimes -- G-computation: parametric estimation of optimal DTRs -- Estimation DTRs for alternative outcome types -- Inference and non-regularity -- Additional considerations and final thoughts. Subjects: Medical statistics. Medical records--Data processing. Statistics as Topic--methods. Data Interpretation, Statistical. Evidence-Based Medicine--methods.

Longitudinal Studies. Models, Statistical. Medical records--Data processing. Medical statistics. Notes: Includes bibliographical references (pages 185-201) and index. Series: Statistics for biology and health, 1431-8776 Statistics for biology and health. 1431-8776 Dewey class no.: 610.72/7 NLM class no.: 2014 A-048 WA 950 National bib agency no.: 101623048 016316998 Other system no.: (OCoLC)ocn830367439 Invalid ISBN: 9781461474289 (ebk.) 1461474280 (ebk.) Content type: text Media type: unmediated Carrier type: volume CALL NUMBER: RA409 .C42 2013 Copy 2 Request in: Jefferson or Adams Building Reading Rooms Shelf Location: FLM2014 031839 CALL NUMBER: RA409 .C42 2013 OVERFLOWA5S Request in: Jefferson or Adams Building Reading Rooms (FLM1)

Statistics for evidence-based practice and evaluation LCCN: 2011944720 Type of material: Book Personal name: Rubin, Allen. Main title: Statistics for evidence-based practice and evaluation/Allen Rubin. Edition: 3rd ed., student ed. Published/Created: Belmont, CA: Brooks/Cole, Cengage Learning, c2013. Description: xvi, 347 p.: ill.; 26 cm. Links: Contributor biographical information http://www.loc.gov/catdir/enhancements/fy1303/2011944720-b.html Publisher description http://www.loc.gov/catdir/enhancements/fy1303/2011944720-d.html Table of contents only http://www.loc.gov/catdir/enhancements/fy1303/2011944720-t.html ISBN: 9780840029140 0840029144 LC classification: RA409 .R83 2013 Subjects: Medical statistics. Evidence-based medicine--Statistical methods. Clinical medicine--Statistical methods. Notes: Includes bibliographical references (p. 339-341) and index. Dewey class no.: 610.72/7 CALL NUMBER: RA409 .R83 2013 Copy 1 Request in: Jefferson or Adams Building Reading Rooms

Stroke prevention, treatment, and rehabilitation LCCN: 2011277797 Type of material: Book Personal name: Spence, J. David. Main title: Stroke prevention, treatment, and rehabilitation/J. David Spence, Henry J.M. Barrett. Published/Created: New York: McGraw-Hill Medical, c2012. Description: xiv, 306 p.: ill.; 23 cm. Links: Publisher description http://www.loc.gov/catdir/enhancements/fy1301/2011277797-d.html Table of contents only http://www.loc.gov/catdir/enhancements/fy1301/2011277797-t.html ISBN: 9780071762359 (alk. paper) 0071762353 (alk. paper) LC classification: RC388.5 .S663 2012 Related names: Barnett, H. J. M. (Henry J. M.) Contents: Importance of stroke and stroke prevention -- Epidemiology of stroke prevention and urgency of treatment -- Potential for stroke prevention -- Preventing stroke -- Nutrition, diabetes, and stroke prevention -- Smoking cessation -- Exercise -- Hypertension -- Antiplatelet therapy -- Anticoagulation -- Lipid-lowering therapy -- Management and prevention of intracranial atherosclerotic disease -- Appropriate endarterectomy and stenting for carotid stenosis -- Finding the cause of the TIA or stroke: the key to appropriate therapy -- Thoughts on the hazards of relying on publications: cautions needed before applying published results to evidence-based medicine -- Prospects for prevention of dementia by prevention of stroke -- Minimizing adverse effects of cardiovascular drugs -- When the stroke wasn't prevented -- Treatment of acute stroke: medical and interventional therapy -- Surgical management of acute stroke -- Stroke rehabilitation. Subjects: Cerebrovascular disease--Prevention. Cerebrovascular disease--Treatment. Cerebrovascular disease--Patients--Rehabilitation. Stroke--prevention & control. Stroke--therapy. Notes: Includes bibliographical references and index. Dewey class no.: 616.81 NLM class no.: 2012 D-894 WL 356 WL 356 S744 2012 National bib agency no.: 101584323 016034520 Other system no.: (OCoLC)ocn748333195 CALL NUMBER: RC388.5 .S663 2012 Copy 1 Request in: Jefferson or Adams Building Reading Rooms

Studying a study & testing a test: reading evidence-based health research LCCN: 2012008446 Type of material: Book Personal name: Riegelman, Richard K. Main title: Studying a study & testing a test: reading evidence-based health research/Richard K. Riegelman. Edition: 6th ed. Published/Created: Philadelphia: Wolters Kluwer/Lippincott Williams & Wilkins Heath, c2013. Description: xii, 338 p.: ill.; 26 cm. ISBN: 9780781774260 (pbk.: alk.

paper) 0781774268 (pbk. alk. paper) LC classification: R118.6 .R54 2013 Variant title: Studying a study and testing a test Related names: Riegelman, Richard K. Studying a study and testing a test Contents: Studying a study: M.A.A.R.I.E. framework, method, assignment, assessment -- Studying a study: M.A.A.R.I.E. framework, results -- Studying a study: M.A.A.R.I.E. framework, interpretation, extrapolation -- Randomized controlled trials -- Observational studies -- Safety - - Meta-analysis -- Testing a test: M.A.A.R.I.E. framework, method, assignment, and assessment -- Testing a test: M.A.A.R.I.E. framework, results, interpretation, extrapolation -- Screening: prediction and decision rules -- Decision and cost-effectiveness analysis: M.A.A.R.I.E. framework, method, assignment, assessment -- Decision and cost-effectiveness analysis: M.A.A.R.I.E. framework, results, interpretation, extrapolation -- A guide to the guidelines -- Translating evidence into practice. Subjects: Medical literature--Evaluation. Medicine--Research--Evaluation. Biometry. Epidemiologic Methods. Evidence-Based Medicine--methods. Notes: Rev. ed. of: Studying a study and testing a test/Richard K. Riegelman. Includes bibliographical references and index. Dewey class no.: 610/.72 NLM class no.: WA 950 Other system no.: (DNLM)101579158 CALL NUMBER: R118.6 .R54 2013 Copy 2 Request in: Jefferson or Adams Building Reading Rooms Shelf Location: FLM2013 000694 CALL NUMBER: R118.6 .R54 2013 OVERFLOWA5S Request in: Jefferson or Adams Building Reading Rooms (FLM1)

Textbook of family medicine LCCN: 2014043849 Type of material: Book Uniform title: Textbook of family practice. Main title: Textbook of family medicine/[edited by] Robert E. Rakel, David P. Rakel. Edition: Ninth edition. Published/Produced: Philadelphia, PA: Elsevier Inc., [2015] Projected pub date: 1504 Description: p.; cm. ISBN: 9780323239905 (hardcover: alk. paper) LC classification: RC46 Related names: Rakel, Robert E., editor. Rakel, David, editor. Subjects: Family Practice. Evidence-Based Medicine. Patient Education as Topic. Notes: Includes bibliographical references and index. Dewey class no.: 610 NLM class no.: WB 110 Other system no.: (DNLM)101645489 Content type: text Media type: unmediated Carrier type: volume

Textbook on evidence-based holistic mind-body medicine: healing the mind in traditional Hippocratic medicine LCCN: 2012939747 Type of material: Book Personal name: Ventegodt, Søren. Main title: Textbook on evidence-based holistic mind-body medicine: healing the mind in traditional Hippocratic medicine/Søren Ventegodt and Joav Merrick. Published/Created: New York: Nova Biomedical: Nova Science Publishers, c2013. Description: xvi, 254 p.: ill.; 26 cm. ISBN: 9781622571123 1622571126 LC classification: R733 .V46 2013 Variant title: Healing the mind in traditional Hippocratic medicine Related names: Merrick, Joav, 1950- Subjects: Holistic medicine. Evidence-based medicine. Mental illness--Treatment. Evidence-based psychiatry. Notes: Includes bibliographical references and index. Series: Health and human development Health and human development. Dewey class no.: 616.891 Other system no.: (OCoLC)ocn859255554 Shelf Location: FLM2014 006053 CALL NUMBER: R733 .V46 2013 OVERFLOWA5S Request in: Jefferson or Adams Building Reading Rooms (FLM1)

Textbook on evidence-based holistic mind-body medicine: holistic practice of traditional Hippocratic medicine LCCN: 2012939753 Type of material: Book Personal name: Ventegodt, Søren, author. Main title: Textbook on evidence-based holistic mind-body medicine: holistic practice of traditional Hippocratic medicine/Søren Ventegodt and Joav Merrick. Published/Produced: New York: Nova Biomedical, [2013] Description: xxvii, 221 pages: illustrations; 26 cm. ISBN: 9781622571055 (hbk.) 1622571053 (hbk.) LC classification: RC49 .V46 2013 Related names: Merrick, Joav, 1950- author. Subjects: Medicine, Psychosomatic. Holistic medicine. Evidence-based medicine. Evidence-based medicine. Holistic medicine. Medicine, Psychosomatic. Notes: Includes bibliographical references and index. Series: Health and human development Health and human development series. Other system no.: (OCoLC)ocn870870469 Content type: text Media type: unmediated Carrier type: volume

Shelf Location: FLM2015 029722 CALL NUMBER: RC49 .V46 2013 OVERFLOWJ34 Request in: Jefferson or Adams Building Reading Rooms (FLM2)

The 5-minute consult clinical companion to women's health LCCN: 2012011795 Type of material: Book Main title: The 5-minute consult clinical companion to women's health/editors, Kelly A. McGarry, Iris L. Tong. Edition: 2nd ed. Published/Created: Philadelphia: Wolters Kluwer/Lippincott Williams & Wilkins Health, c2013. Description: xiii, 261 p.; 28 cm. ISBN: 9781451116540 (hardback) 1451116543 (hardback) LC classification: RC48.6 .A13 2013 Variant title: Five-minute consult clinical companion to women's health Portion of title Clinical companion to women's health Related names: McGarry, Kelly A. Tong, Iris L. Summary: "The 5-Minute Consult Clinical Companion to Women's Health is a quick-reference guide to the diagnosis and management of symptoms and disorders that commonly occur in women. Written by both primary care physicians and obstetrician-gynecologists, the book covers disorders that are unique to women, occur disproportionately in women, or have a different clinical presentation, course, and/or prognosis in women. The contributors present practical, up-to-date, evidence-based information in a format designed for rapid consultation"--Provided by publisher. Subjects: Women's Health--Handbooks. Evidence-Based Medicine--Handbooks. Notes: Includes bibliographical references and index. Series: 5-minute consult Dewey class no.: 613/.04244 NLM class no.: WA 39 Other system no.: (DNLM)101580644 Shelf Location: FLM2014 182494 CALL NUMBER: RC48.6 .A13 2013 OVERFLOWA5S Request in: Jefferson or Adams Building Reading Rooms (FLM1)

The AIDS conspiracy: science fights back LCCN: 2011045297 Type of material: Book Personal name: Nattrass, Nicoli. Main title: The AIDS conspiracy: science fights back/Nicoli Nattrass. Published/Created: New York: Columbia University Press, c2012. Projected pub date: 1202 Description: p.; cm. ISBN: 9780231149129 (cloth: alk. paper) 9780231520256 (ebook) Contents: The conspiratorial move against HIV science and its consequences -- AIDS origin conspiracy theories in the United States and South Africa -- Who believes AIDS conspiracy theories and why leadership matters -- Science, politics, and credibility: David Gilbert fights AIDS conspiracy beliefs in US prisons -- Science, conspiracy theory, and the South African AIDS policy tragedy -- Hero scientists, cultropreneurs, living icons, and praise-singers: AIDS denialism as community -- Defending the imprimatur of science: Duesberg and the medical hypotheses saga -- The conspiratorial move and the struggle for evidence-based medicine. Subjects: HIV Infections--South Africa. HIV Infections--United States. Acquired Immunodeficiency Syndrome--South Africa. Acquired Immunodeficiency Syndrome--United States. Health Policy--South Africa. Health Policy--United States. Public Opinion--South Africa. Public Opinion--United States. Notes: Includes bibliographical references and index. Dewey class no.: 362.196/9792 NLM class no.: WC 503 Other system no.: (DNLM)101572093

The AIDS conspiracy: science fights back LCCN: 2012435459 Type of material: Book Personal name: Nattrass, Nicoli. Main title: The AIDS conspiracy: science fights back/Nicoli Nattrass. Published/Produced: Johannesburg: Wits University Press, 2012. Description: viii, 225 pages: illustrations; 24 cm ISBN: 9781868145621 (paperback) 186814562X (paperback) LC classification: RA644.A25 N297 2012 Contents: The conspiratorial move against HIV science and its consequences -- AIDS origin conspiracy theories in the United States and South Africa -- Who believes AIDS conspiracy theories and why leadership matters -- Science, politics, and credibility: David Gilbert fights AIDS conspiracy beliefs in US prisons -- Science, conspiracy theory, and the South African AIDS policy tragedy -- Hero scientists, cultropreneurs, living icons, and praise-singers: AIDS denialism as community -- Defending the imprimatur of science: Duesberg and the medical hypotheses saga -- The conspiratorial move and the struggle for evidence-based medicine. Subjects: AIDS (Disease)--Transmission. HIV infections--United States. HIV infections--South Africa. Conspiracy theories. AIDS (Disease)--United States. AIDS (Disease)--South Africa. Public opinion--United States. Public opinion--South Africa. Notes: Includes bibliographical references (pages [193]-216) and index. Dewey class no.: 362.1969792 Other system no.: (OCoLC)ocn809000675 Content type: text Media type: unmediated Carrier type: volume Shelf Location: FLM2013 000363 CALL NUMBER: RA644.A25 N297 2012 OVERFLOWA5S Request in: Jefferson or Adams Building Reading Rooms (FLM1)

The evidence-based guide to antidepressant medications LCCN: 2011032536 Type of material: Book Main title: The evidence-based guide to antidepressant medications/edited by Anthony J. Rothschild. Edition: 1st ed. Published/Created: Washington, DC: American Psychiatric Pub., c2012. Description: xix, 404 p.: ill.; 23 cm. ISBN: 9781585624058 (pbk.: alk. paper) LC classification: RM332 .E95 2012 Related names: Rothschild, Anthony J. American Psychiatric Association. Contents: Unipolar and bipolar depression -- Anxiety disorders/Ryan J. Kimmel, Peter P. Roy-Byrne -- Schizophrenia and schizoaffective disorder/Deepak Cyril D'Souza, Rajiv Radhakrshnan -- Personality disorders/Kenneth R. Silk, Michael D. Jibson -- Substance-related disorders/Avram H. Mack -- Use of antidepressant medications in children and adolescents/Mary S. Ahn, Lauren Yakutis, Jean A. Frazier -- Use of antidepressant medications in the geriatric patient/Benjamin Liptzin, Cassandra Hobgood -- Use of antidepressants in the medically ill/Stacey B. Gramann, Nancy Byatt -- Use of antidepressants during pregnancy and lactation/Kristina M. Deligiannidis -- Evidenced based nursing care of patients prescribed antidepressants/Judith Shindul-Rothschild. Subjects: Mental Disorders--drug therapy. Antidepressive Agents--therapeutic use. Evidence-Based Medicine--methods. Notes: Includes bibliographical references and index. Dewey class no.: 616.85/27061 Other system no.: (DNLM)101565852 CALL NUMBER: RM332 .E95 2012 Copy 1 Request in: Jefferson or Adams Building Reading Rooms CALL NUMBER: RM332 .E95 2012 LANDOVR Copy 2 Request in: Jefferson or Adams Building Reading Rooms - STORED OFFSITE

The organization of critical care: an evidence-based approach to improving quality LCCN: 2014940928 Type of material: Book Main title: The organization of critical care: an evidence-based approach to improving quality/Damon C. Scales, Gordon D. Rubenfeld, editors. Published/Produced: New York: Humana Press, [2014] ©2014 Description: ix, 284 pages: illustrations; 24 cm ISBN: 9781493908103 (alk. paper) 1493908103 (alk. paper) LC classification: RC86.7 .O73 2014 Related names: Scales, Damon C. (Damon Cole), 1971- editor. Rubenfeld, Gordon D., editor. Subjects: Critical care medicine. Critical Care--organization & administration. Evidence-Based Medicine. Quality Improvement. Notes: Includes bibliographical references (some color) and index. Series: Respiratory medicine, 2197-7372 Respiratory medicine (New York, N.Y.) 2197-7372 Dewey class no.: 616.02/8 NLM class no.: 2014 K-576 WX 218 National bib agency no.: 101642354 Other system no.: (OCoLC)ocn888996191 Invalid ISBN: 9781493908110 (eBook) 1493908111 (eBook) Content type: text Media type: unmediated Carrier type: volume Shelf Location: FLM2015 062860 CALL NUMBER: RC86.7 .O73 2014 OVERFLOWJ34 Request in: Jefferson or Adams Building Reading Rooms (FLM2)

The Oxford handbook of evidence-based management LCCN: 2011036150 Type of material: Book Main title: The Oxford handbook of evidence-based management/edited by Denise M. Rousseau. Published/Created: New York: Oxford University Press, 2012. Description: xxviii, 432 p.: ill.; 26 cm. ISBN: 9780199763986 (acid-free paper) 0199763984 (acid-free paper) LC classification: HD30.23 .O955 2012 Related names: Rousseau, Denise M. Contents: Envisioning evidence-based management/Denise M. Rousseau -- Learning from other evidence-based practices: the case of medicine/E.G.R. Barends, Steven ten Have & Franck Huisman -- A design science approach to evidence-based management/J.E. Van Aken & A.G.L. Romme -- Organizational behavior's contributions to evidence-based management/Denise M. Rousseau -- Evidence-based management in "macro" organizational theory and strategy/Ravi Madhavan & Joseph T. Mahoney -- Evidence-based entrepreneurship (EBE): a systematic approach to cumulative science/Michael Frese ... [et al.] -- Systematic review and evidence synthesis as a practice and scholarship tool/Rob Briner & David Denyer -- Research findings practitioners resist: lessons for management academics from evidence-based medicine/Tamara Giluk & Sara L. Rynes -- Enabling evidence-based management: bridging the gap between academics and practitioners/Opal Leung & Jean Bartunek -- Adventures in the evidence-based management trade/Anthony Kovner -- At the intersection of the academy and practice at asbury heights/John Zanardelli -- Evidence-based decision management/Frank J. Yates & Georges Potwoworski -- Decision logic in evidence-based management: can standard business logical models make managers better human resource decision makers?/John W. Boudreau -- EBMgt and organizational facts/Lex Donaldson -- Buried treasure: finding evidence now/Roye Werner -- Culture and evidence-based management/Georges Potwoworski & Lee Green -- Designing EBMgt implementation processes and practices for the senior management, middle management and supervisor levels/Jayne Speicher-Bocija & Richard Adams -- Teaching and learning using evidence-based principles/Jodi Goodman & James O'Brien -- Teaching and learning evidence-based management 1.0/Blake Jelley, Wendy R. Carroll & Denise M. Rousseau -- Toward doctoral education that encourages evidence-based management through problem-focused research/Paul Salipante & Ann K. Smith -- Creating evidence-based management textbooks/Jone L. Pearce -- Beyond "new scientific management"--why the ideological critique of evidence-based management should be taken seriously/Severin Hornung -- The politics of evidence-based decision making/Gerard P. Hodgkinson. Subjects: Decision making. Business intelligence. Management. Series: Oxford library of psychology Dewey class no.: 658.4/03 CALL NUMBER: HD30.23 .O955 2012 Copy 1 Request in: Jefferson or Adams Building Reading Rooms CALL NUMBER: HD30.23 .O955 2012 Copy 2 Request in:

Jefferson or Adams Building Reading Rooms

The practice of cognitive-behavioural hypnotherapy: a manual for evidence-based clinical hypnosis LCCN: 2013427133 Type of material: Book Personal name: Robertson, Donald, 1972- Main title: The practice of cognitive-behavioural hypnotherapy: a manual for evidence-based clinical hypnosis/Donald J. Robertson. Published/Created: London: Karnac, 2013. Description: xiii, 444 p.: ill.; 24 cm. ISBN: 9781855755307 (pbk.) 1855755300 (pbk.) LC classification: RC497 .R63 2013 Subjects: Hypnotism--Therapeutic use. Cognitive therapy. Hypnosis. Cognitive Therapy. Evidence-Based Medicine--methods. Notes: Includes bibliographical references and index. Dewey class no.: 615.8/512 NLM class no.: 2013 A-877 WM 415 National bib agency no.: 101601410 Other system no.: (OCoLC)ocn824849408 Shelf Location: FLM2014 002995 CALL NUMBER: RC497 .R63 2013 OVERFLOWA5S Request in: Jefferson or Adams Building Reading Rooms (FLM1)

The vitamin cure for depression LCCN: 2012038641 Type of material: Book Personal name: Jonsson, Bo H., 1950- Main title: The vitamin cure for depression/Bo H. Jonsson, M.D., Ph.D. and Andrew W. Saul, Ph.D. Published/Produced: Laguna Beach, CA: Basic Health Publications, Inc., [2012] Description: xix, 220 pages: illustrations; 22 cm ISBN: 9781591202820 (alk. paper) LC classification: RC537 .J67 2012 Related names: Saul, Andrew W. Contents: The plague of depression -- An evolutionary view of depression -- Conventional treatment and traditional science -- Evidence-based medicine: neither good evidence nor good medicine -- Orthomolecular medicine and biochemical individuality -- An evolution-based health program -- Food really does matter -- Orthomolecular treatment -- Multinutrient treatment -- Bipolar disorder -- In the now -- Unstress and un-depress your life -- Depression: observations and comments -- Case histories. Subjects: Depression, Mental--Chemotherapy. Vitamin therapy. Notes: Includes bibliographical references (pages 183-185) and index. Dewey class no.: 616.85/27061 Content type: text Media type: unmediated Carrier type: volume CALL NUMBER: RC537 .J67 2012 Copy 1 Request in: Jefferson or Adams Building Reading Rooms

Therapeutic electrophysical agents: evidence behind practice LCCN: 2013035769 Type of material: Book Personal name: Bélanger, Alain, author. Main title: Therapeutic electrophysical agents: evidence behind practice/Alain-Yvan Bélanger, PhD, PT, Retired Professor, Laval University, Canada, owner and consultant, Physiométrix Inc. Edition: Third edition. Published/Produced: Philadelphia: Wolters Kluwer/Lippincott Williams & Wilkins Health, [2014] ©2014 Description: xiii, 434 pages: color illustrations; 28 cm ISBN: 9781451182743 (pbk.) 1451182740 (pbk.) LC classification: RM841.5 .B45 2014 Contents: Therapeutic electrophysical agents in health care -- Toward a practice based on evidence -- Soft-tissue healing process -- Pain following soft-tissue pathology -- Purchase, electrical safety, and maintenance -- Therapeutic spectrum, selection and indication -- Thermotherapy -- Cryotherapy -- Hydrotherapy -- Shortwave diathermy -- Low-level laser therapy -- Ultraviolet -- Neuromuscular electrical stimulation -- Transcutaneous electrical nerve stimulation -- Electrical stimulation for tissue healing and repair -- Iontophoresis -- Spinal traction -- Limb compression -- Continuous passive motion -- Ultrasound -- Extracorporeal shock wave therapy. Subjects: Therapeutics--Handbooks. Therapeutics--Outlines. Evidence-Based Medicine--Handbooks. Evidence-Based Medicine--Outlines. Physical and Rehabilitation Medicine--Handbooks. Physical and Rehabilitation Medicine--Outlines. Notes: Includes bibliographical references and index. Dewey class no.: 615.8/3 NLM class no.: WB 39 Other system no.: (DNLM)101616271 Content type: text Media type: unmediated Carrier type: volume Shelf Location: FLM2014 199962 CALL NUMBER: RM841.5 .B45 2014 OVERFLOWA5S Request in: Jefferson or Adams Building Reading Rooms (FLM1)

Trigger point dry needling: an evidence and clinical-based approach LCCN: 2014451679 Type of material: Book Main title: Trigger point dry needling: an evidence and clinical-based approach/edited by Jan

Dommerholt, DPT, DPT, MPS, Myopain Seminars, LLC, Bethesda Physicians, Inc., Bethesda, Maryland, USA, Universidad CEU Cardenal Herrera, Valencia, Spain, Shenandoah University, Winchester, VA, USA, and César Fernández-de-las-Peñas, PT, DO, PhD, Department of Physical Therapy, Occupational Therapy, Physical Medicine and Rehabilitation of Universidad Rey Juan Carlos, Alcorón, Madrid, Spain, Ethesiology Laboratory of Universidad Rey Juan Carlos, Alcorón, Madrid, Spain, and, Centre for Sensory-Motor Interaction (SMI), Department of Health Science and Technology, Aalborg University, Aalborg, Denmark,; forewords by Leon Chaitow, ND, DO (UK), Registered Osteopath and Naturopath, Honororary Fellow and Former Senior Lecturer, School of Life Sciences, University of Westminister, London, UK, Fellow, British Naturopathic Association, and Robert D. Gerwin, MD, Associate Professor, Department of Neurology at Johns Hopkins University School of Medicine, Baltimore, Maryland, USA, President, Pain & Rehabilitation Medicine, Bethesda, Maryland, USA. Published/Produced: Edinburgh; New York: Churchill Livingstone/Elsevier, 2013. Description: xviii, 258 pages: illustrations; 26 cm ISBN: 9780702046018 (hbk.) 0702046019 (hbk.) LC classification: RC927.3 .T75 2013 Related names: Dommerholt, Jan, editor. Fernández-de-las-Peñas, César, editor. Subjects: Myofascial pain syndromes--Treatment. Acupuncture. Myofascial Pain Syndromes--therapy. Acupuncture Therapy. Evidence-Based Medicine. Trigger Points. Notes: Includes bibliographical references and index. NLM class no.: 2013 C-609 WE 550 National bib no.: GBB2B1714 National bib agency no.: 101605493 016205369 Other system no.: (OCoLC)ocn817257742 Content type: text Media type: unmediated Carrier type: volume CALL NUMBER: RC927.3 .T75 2013 Copy 1 Request in: Jefferson or Adams Building Reading Rooms

Tumor board review: guideline and case reviews in oncology LCCN: 2014040453 Type of material: Book Main title: Tumor board review: guideline and case reviews in oncology/editors, Robert F. Todd, III, Kathleen A. Cooney,

Teresa G. Hayes, Martha Pritchett Mims, Francis P. Worden. Edition: Second edition. Published/Produced: New York: Demos Medical, [2015] Projected pub date: 1501 Description: p.; cm. ISBN: 9781620700600 LC classification: RC254 Related names: Todd, Robert F., III, editor. Cooney, Kathleen A., editor. Hayes, Teresa G., editor. Mims, Martha Pritchett, editor. Worden, Francis P., editor. Subjects: Neoplasms--Case Reports. Neoplasms--Practice Guideline. Evidence-Based Medicine--Case Reports. Evidence-Based Medicine--Practice Guideline. Notes: Includes bibliographical references and index. Dewey class no.: 616.99/4 NLM class no.: QZ 200 Other system no.: (DNLM)101643323 Invalid ISBN: 9781617052231 (e-book) Content type: text Media type: unmediated Carrier type: volume

Tumor board reviews: guidelines and case reviews in oncology LCCN: 2011036095 Type of material: Book Main title: Tumor board reviews: guidelines and case reviews in oncology/editors, Robert F. Todd III ... [et al.]. Published/Created: New York, NY: Demos Medical Pub., c2012. Description: xi, 363 p.: ill.; 29 cm. ISBN: 9781936287178 (alk. paper) 9781617050466 (e-book) LC classification: RC254 .T85 2012 Related names: Todd, Robert F. Subjects: Tumors--Case Reports. Tumors--Practice Guideline. Evidence-based medicine--Case Reports. Evidence-based medicine--Practice Guideline. Notes: Includes bibliographical references and index. Dewey class no.: 616.99/4 Other system no.: (DNLM)101567867 CALL NUMBER: RC254 .T85 2012 Copy 1 Request in: Jefferson or Adams Building Reading Rooms

Understanding value-based healthcare LCCN: 2014046528 Type of material: Book Main title: Understanding value-based healthcare/editors, Christopher Moriates, Vineet Arora, Neel Shah. Published/Produced: New York: McGraw-Hill, 2015. Projected pub date: 1506 Description: p.; cm. ISBN: 9780071816984 (alk. paper) 0071816984 (alk. paper) LC classification: RA410 Related names: Moriates, Christopher, 1982-, editor. Arora, Vineet, editor. Shah, Neel (Obstetrician/Gynecologist), editor. Contents: The current state of healthcare costs and waste in the United States --

Medical coverage in the United States -- The challenges of understanding healthcare pricing -- Defining value: connecting quality and safety to the costs of care -- A changing landscape: cost consciousness and value in healthcare delivery -- Ethics of cost conscious care -- The importance of zip codes and genetic codes: variation in resource utilization -- Stents, robots, and the role of technology diffusion -- Primary care shortage crisis: lost opportunities to deliver value/David Margolius and Andrew Morris-Singer -- Barriers to providing high-value care/Daisy Smith and Steven Weinberger -- Building a pipeline for change: teaching about cost awareness and evidence-based medicine -- The role of patients: shared decision making, e-patients, and consumer directed healthcare -- High-value medication prescribing -- Screening and prevention: balancing benefits with harms and costs -- Shifting incentives: moving reimbursement from volume to value -- Implementing value-based initiatives: a new challenge for clinicians and healthcare systems. Subjects: Delivery of Health Care--economics--United States--Case Reports. Costs and Cost Analysis--United States--Case Reports. Economics, Medical--United States--Case Reports. Notes: Includes bibliographical references and index. Dewey class no.: 338.4/73621 NLM class no.: W 84 AA1 Other system no.: (DNLM)101647360 Content type: text Media type: unmediated Carrier type: volume

Users' guides to the medical literature. A manual for evidence-based clinical practice LCCN: 2014031343 Type of material: Book Main title: Users' guides to the medical literature. A manual for evidence-based clinical practice/[edited by] Gordon Guyatt, Drummond Rennie, Maureen O. Meade, Deborah J. Cook. Edition: Third edition. Published/Produced: New York: McGraw-Hill Education Medical, [2015] Projected pub date: 1410 Description: p.; cm. ISBN: 9780071790710 (paperback: alk. paper) 0071790713 (paperback: alk. paper) LC classification: R723.7 Variant title: Manual for evidence-based clinical practice Related names: Guyatt, Gordon, editor. Rennie, Drummond, editor. Meade, Maureen, editor. Cook, Deborah, 1960-, editor. American Medical Association. JAMA & archives. Subjects:

Evidence-Based Medicine--Resource Guides. Clinical Medicine--Resource Guides. Decision Making--Resource Guides. Review Literature as Topic--Resource Guides. Notes: Preceded by: Users' guides to the medical literature/the Evidence-Based Medicine Working Group; editors, Gordon Guyatt ... [et al.]. 2nd ed. 2008. "JAMA & Archives Journals." Includes bibliographical references and index. Series: JAMAevidence JAMAevidence. Dewey class no.: 610 NLM class no.: WB 39 Other system no.: (DNLM)101638774 Content type: text Media type: unmediated Carrier type: volume

Users' guides to the medical literature. Essentials of evidence-based clinical practice LCCN: 2014031341 Type of material: Book Main title: Users' guides to the medical literature. Essentials of evidence-based clinical practice/[edited by] Gordon Guyatt, Drummond Rennie, Marueen O. Meade, Deborah J. Cook. Edition: Third edition. Published/Produced: New York: McGraw-Hill Education Medical, [2015] Projected pub date: 1410 Description: p.; cm. ISBN: 9780071794152 (pbk.: alk. paper) 0071794158 (pbk.: alk. paper) LC classification: RC46 Variant title: Essentials of evidence-based clinical practice Related titles: Abridgement of (work): Users' guides to the medial literature. A manual for evidence-based clinical practice. Related names: Guyatt, Gordon, editor. Rennie, Drummond, editor. Meade, Maureen, editor. Cook, Deborah, 1960-, editor. Summary: "The streamlined companion to the classic Users' guides to the medical literature--fully updated and revised. This compact guide condenses the most clinically relevant content of the landmark Users' Guides to the Medical Literature to help you incorporate evidence-based medicine into your practice. You will learn the principles of evidence-based medicine, how your practice can benefit from the constant stream of new medical literature, and how to differentiate good medical evidence from bad. This edition includes several new chapters and a new emphasis on the role of patient preferences and preappraised resources.--Provided by publisher. Subjects: Evidence-Based Medicine. Clinical Medicine. Decision Making. Review Literature as Topic. Notes: Preceded by Users' guides to the medical literature: the essentials of evidence-based clinical practice/the Evidence-Based Medicine Working Group; editors, Gordon Guyatt ... [et al.]. 2nd ed. 2008. Abridgement of Users' guides to the medical literature. A manual for evidence-based clinical practice. Third edition. 2015. "JAMA & Archives Journals." Includes bibliographical references and index. Dewey class no.: 616 NLM class no.: WB 102.5 Other system no.: (DNLM)101638810 Content type: text Media type: unmediated Carrier type: volume

Index

B

C

D

E

F

G

H

M

N

O

P

Q

R

S

T

U

V

W

Y